HEALTH
FIRST

HEALTH FIRST

Winning at Weight Loss and Wellness

Steve Hirsch, MD

Foreword by Robert Steiner
Afterword by Kathy Stewart

Toronto and New York

Published in 2013 by
BPS Books
Toronto & New York
www.bpsbooks.com
A division of Bastian Publishing Services Ltd.

ISBN 978-1-927483-53-4

Cataloguing-in-Publication Data available from Library
and Archives Canada.

Cover: Gnibel
Text design and typesetting: Daniel Crack, Kinetics Design, www.kdbooks.ca

Contents

Foreword

A Conversation That Changed My Life

It is no exaggeration to say that in just one very clear twenty-minute conversation, Dr. Steve Hirsch changed the way I live my life. He did so in four ways.

First, by drawing attention to the "small" bulge I was getting used to; I was almost in the obesity category, he said. Other doctors had missed that entirely, or had simply accepted that this is what happens to a man in his early forties.

Second, by making me pay attention to the way I eat, every time I eat. No tricks or special foods. Just very conscious portioning on a weekly basis. As long as I was eating well, and in proportion, I could eat whenever I was hungry. The key, he taught me, was to be mindful about when I was actually hungry.

Third, by showing me how I could incorporate exercise into my weekly routine. Nothing huge or ambitious. Just forty-five minutes three times a week, which I adapted to thirty minutes five times a week to fit my schedule.

And finally, by showing me how to measure my progress every day. Two pounds a week, week after week. Nothing radical. Just steady.

Four years later, I have kept most of the weight off. I am grateful every day for that conversation in his office.

As more and more of us stand on the threshold of diabetes,

heart disease, stroke, and the simple unpleasantness of being too heavy, this book puts Dr. Hirsch in everyone's hands, so anyone, anywhere, can benefit from the kind of conversation that helped me so much.

As a journalism educator, I try to help specialists communicate new ideas very clearly – so they deepen our understanding of the world around us. Health can be very complicated. But Dr. Hirsch does what every doctor should: he truly puts our health in our own hands.

–*ROBERT STEINER, Director, Fellowships in Global Journalism,*
Munk School of Global Affairs, University of Toronto

Acknowledgments

Writing this book was a dream of mine for a number of years. However, it was only after reading *The Success Principles*, written by Jack Canfield, that I drew the inspiration to just lean into it and get started on this "breakthrough goal." Thank you so much, Jack, for motivating me to begin writing.

My dear friend Sheryl Shapiro provided me with the name of a writer, Donna Green, who helped me translate my Health First program from clinical practice to text. Donna was instrumental in working with me, chapter by chapter, to develop the first draft of the manuscript. Her commitment and dedication to this project not only helped me transform my concepts and ideas into text but also kept me on track with deadlines. Thank you, Donna, for your incredible help and hard work.

My wife, Paula, was a tremendous support in so many ways throughout this entire project. She encouraged me to stick with it when the going got tough, and provided invaluable feedback, editing, and suggestions for change at every stage of the process. Thank you, Paula, from the bottom of my heart, for your ongoing and unwavering support.

My two sons, Jason and Neil, encouraged me to write this book over many years. Their ongoing enthusiasm was a continual source of inspiration for me. Guys, thank you so much.

Lorne Greenspan, a friend and colleague, was very supportive during the writing process. He encouraged me to persevere when challenges arose and was always very supportive. Lorne, thank you.

In July 2012, with three or four chapters left to write, I was feeling stuck. I applied and was accepted to a retreat in Hawaii with Jack Canfield, Stewart and Joan Emery, and seventeen other wonderful participants from around the world. We spent five days together, working on our personal goals and helping one another to achieve a breakthrough goal. Jack, Stewart, and Joan, thank you so much for your guidance and support. Your valuable lessons helped propel me to the next level. Additionally, my fellow participants provided me with tremendous encouragement and the determination necessary to continue writing. To Ian Bailey, Aleesa Daley, Kathy Davenport, Marc Gottlieb, Erika Labansat, Tatiana and Mykola Latansky, Katja Narva, Guillermo Paz, Natalie Peace, Marc Pletzer, Lewis Pugh, Ellis Rubenstein, Patrick Ryan, Kelly Shorter, Kristi Staab, and Stewart Welch, thank you all so much. And to Alice Doughty and Patty Aubery with The Jack Canfield Companies, thank you for your support and enthusiasm for this book during the retreat and over the subsequent months.

Following completion of the first draft, several colleagues and friends kindly and enthusiastically agreed to conduct a review of the manuscript for me. Each of you provided me with excellent feedback and suggestions for improvement. I greatly appreciate the time and effort that you all devoted to the review. Thank you to my dear friends Diana Brecher and Diane Davies, to my colleagues Arielle Cheifetz and Jennifer Brighton, and to my brother-in-law and closest friend, Mark Adler.

To my colleague and mentor Cal Gutkin, thank you for reviewing the final manuscript, and for your advice and excellent comments. I greatly appreciate the time you spent on this.

When it came time to add the graphics, my close friend Gavin Herman recommended me to Irwin Milgrom of Milgrom and Associates, who were fantastic. Irwin, thank you for your great interest in this book, and for the help of your photographer Larry

Mead. Larry, thank you so very much for your time, tremendous patience, and great work.

Finally, when it came time to find a publisher, my friend, Cy Charney, an accomplished author, put me in touch with Don Bastian, of Bastian Publishing Services. Don, it has been terrific working with you. Your editorial suggestions have been of tremendous help and your relentless commitment to ensuring a high quality standard is greatly appreciated. Thank you so much for your guidance and for your helpful editing – as well as that of your assistant, Monica Kanellis – and for the wonderful artistic text design provided by your designer, Daniel Crack.

Introduction

Life is not a dress rehearsal. Each of us gets only one life. Many things that we hope to enjoy and that we dream of require good health. You can decrease your odds of getting many common chronic diseases that can significantly affect the quality and duration of your life by taking control and acting *now* to prevent disease.

I have helped many patients achieve lifestyle changes – weight loss, increased physical activity, and exercise – all of which help prevent chronic diseases. These include diabetes, heart disease, high cholesterol, pre-diabetes, osteoarthritis, certain cancers, and Alzheimer's disease. For patients who already have diseases, the program has improved their health – in many cases eliminating or reducing their need for medication.

From the day I entered medical practice in 1983, the most rewarding part of my practice, the part I've been most passionate about and that has been the most gratifying, is helping patients achieve and sustain lifestyle changes to improve and prevent so many of the diseases currently plaguing our society. Helping my patients lose significant amounts of weight and embrace exercise and physical activity as a part of their lives has inspired me. Their success has motivated me to continue my quest to prevent chronic disease by sharing my knowledge and expertise with you, through this book.

My recipe for success, shared in these pages, is simple and easy to follow. I call it the Health First program. It's about improving your health and decreasing your risk of developing many chronic diseases. Many of my patients have told me that this program is the first one they've tried that has actually worked for them over the long term. I'm confident that you, too, will be successful if you follow the program. Do this for yourself. Give yourself a gift – the best odds possible for a quality life.

Through the tools provided in this book, you will address the challenge of losing weight and will incorporate physical activity and exercise into your life. This will allow you to achieve your goal of permanent weight loss, the first step to a life of wellness. Your success will truly transform your life. You, too, can become a role model and an ambassador of good health. You can join me and others in halting the world's obesity pandemic, one person at a time.

As you take this journey with me, I believe you'll be inspired by the stories I share of patients who have transformed their lives through committing to these simple tools. They have learned through this journey that it's not just about weight, it's about health and wellness.

The Journey Ahead

Here's a preview of the journey of this book.

The first chapter looks at the bad news about obesity, poor eating habits, and lack of exercise, and the good news of how these problems can be counteracted. The second chapter promotes the attitude and practice of becoming mindful of food choices and consumption. Chapters three and four (a) explore the food groups and their benefits and dangers, as the case may be; (b) present daily "budgets" to follow regarding the food you eat; and (c) present easy-to-develop – and follow – meal plans.

Then come two drill-down chapters on sugar and the deadly duo of fat and salt. The book ends with chapters on physical activity and exercise and how to maintain your new healthy lifestyle.

A Note About Patient Stories

The patient stories included in this book are all true. My patients generously gave me their permission to use their stories; nevertheless, to protect confidentiality, I have withheld their real names and occasionally changed their age and gender. Though they remain anonymous in print, I extend my heartfelt gratitude to them for their support of this book.

A Note About Scientific Information

The information in this book is accurate at the time of writing. However, as you read, keep in mind that new studies are reported daily (some of them being scientifically rigorous and others not), so what seems scientifically proven today may change tomorrow, given new information.

1

It's Your Health:

···

Taking Back Control

People become really quite remarkable when they start thinking they can do things. When they believe in themselves, they have the first secret of success.

−Norman Vincent Peale

This is a bad news/good news chapter. It looks at the threats to our health in our society today and how I have developed my Health First program to deal with them.

The Bad News

Obesity has become a major, worldwide health problem. Whether in Canada, the United States, the UK, Australia, or many other countries, the number of people who are either significantly over-weight or obese is daunting. As you know, there is a dramatic increase in type 2 diabetes worldwide. In the vast majority of cases, the cause is significant weight gain or obesity.

Many people are unaware of the long list of diseases directly related to obesity. According to the Centers for Disease Prevention and Control, obesity substantially increases the risk of the following conditions:

• Coronary heart disease, stroke, and high blood pressure

- Type 2 diabetes
- Cancers, such as endometrial, breast, and colon cancer
- High total cholesterol, or high levels of triglycerides
- Liver and gallbladder disease
- Sleep apnea and respiratory problems
- Degeneration of cartilage and underlying bone within a joint (osteoarthritis)
- Reproductive health complications, such as infertility
- Mental health conditions[*]

If a list of these illnesses isn't motivational enough, let's take a look at the consequences of developing the most prevalent of these: type 2 diabetes.

Type 2 diabetes is the leading cause of adult blindness, kidney failure, and leg amputation. Statistics compiled by the American Diabetes Association reveal that adults with diabetes die from heart disease two to four times more frequently than adults without diabetes. The risk of stroke among diabetics is also two to four times higher than for the non-diabetic population.

Being Sedentary

According to the National Cancer Institute, lack of physical activity is a proven risk factor for breast cancer. It is also implicated in colon cancer and prostate cancer.[†]

Those who are sedentary are also more likely to have higher blood pressure than those who are physically active and exercise regularly. And, as many of you know, the majority of strokes are caused by high blood pressure.

Poor Diet

Our food is too rich in bad fats, sugar, and starches. Diseases linked to diet cause three out of every four deaths in America. These diseases include heart disease, high blood pressure, stroke, some

---

[*] Source: Centers for Disease Control and Prevention <http://www.cdc.gov/chronic disease/resources/publications/AAG/obesity.htm> (1/5/12).

[†] <http://www.cancer.gov/cancertopics/factsheet/prevention/physicalactivity> (1/5/12).

types of cancers, and type 2 diabetes. However, eating a diet that contains five to nine servings of fruits and vegetables a day as part of a healthy, active lifestyle can lower your risk of getting any of these diseases.*

Even if you're not overweight, a poor diet can result in high cholesterol, and this can lead to heart disease and stroke. These two diseases also increase the risk of dementia.

One of the more alarming realities is that doctors are now seeing an increase in the number of children and adolescents with type 2 diabetes due to obesity. A key insight, not generally acknowledged yet critical to the fight against childhood obesity, is role modeling by parents. Studies have clearly shown that, in most cases, when parents are at a healthy weight, are physically active, and exercise regularly, their children follow suit and are not overweight or obese.

The Health First program is aimed at adults, but it can also be used by those who are in their late teens.

You've heard it a million times before: Eat less and exercise more.

So … why don't we? Maybe it's because it seems too hard. Food portions have become excessive, both in restaurants and in packaged goods on grocery store shelves. Many people complain that they don't have enough time to exercise due to the hectic pace of their lives. It is also common for people to reject the idea that anything can happen to them until they are faced with a diagnosis of pre-diabetes, high blood pressure, or high cholesterol.

Many of my patients, still free from disease but with a body mass index (BMI) in the obesity category or in the high end of the overweight category, understood their risks and embraced the Health First program to prevent lifestyle diseases from ever affecting them.

Creating the motivation to do something about poor lifestyle is the first challenge I address through the Health First program. I'd like to walk you through the following simple exercise.

---

* Source: National Cancer Institute <http://www.cancer.gov/search/results> (1.5.12).

Think of people nearest to you who have a chronic health condition (this can include you). Using their names, list each person's illness.

Name: Illness:

_____   _____

_____   _____

_____   _____

_____   _____

_____   _____

What did you find? I'm willing to bet you identified heart disease, diabetes, osteoarthritis, stroke, breast and colon cancer, and Alzheimer's disease on your list. These are among today's most common diseases. If you're either in the high-end overweight or the obesity categories on the BMI measurement tool (see BMI chart, pages 12 and 13) and are not physically active, your risk of getting these illnesses is significantly increased.

For some individuals, genetic factors may figure in the etiology (causation) of these diseases, but genetic history does not always predict disease destiny. By choosing a healthier lifestyle, you can significantly reduce your risk of getting these diseases, even if your genes make you more susceptible to them.

The Good News

But here's the good news: Following the Health First program will dramatically reduce your risk of today's most prevalent lifestyle diseases.

If you need to lose weight and already have …

- **Type 2 diabetes**, it will help you significantly improve your blood sugars and reduce your risk of developing the complications of the disease

- **High blood pressure** related to lifestyle choices, it will help you lower your blood pressure and, in some cases, allow you to reduce or stop your blood pressure medication for good (but only under your own doctor's supervision)

- **Osteoarthritis**, it has the potential to diminish your pain and possibly reduce your future need for hip or knee replacements
- **Breast cancer**, it will decrease your chances of recurrence

The Health First program is not a magic pill, but success is easier than you think. By following the program as outlined in this book, you'll be healthier, dramatically reduce your risk of getting many diseases, and feel revitalized.

This is not just another diet book. The Health First program is not just about weight loss – it's about your health. With so much riding on your health, I believe you owe it to yourself and those who love you to transform your life, one step at a time. My patients – regardless of age – have done it, and you can, too.

According to the National Cancer Institute, people in the obesity category are at increased risk for the following cancers:

- Esophageal
- Pancreatic
- Colon and Rectal
- Breast (after menopause)
- Endometrial (lining of the uterus)
- Kidney
- Thyroid
- Gallbladder

The Next Steps for You

Why do you want to lose weight?

- Is it to decrease your risk of developing a particular disease?
- Is it to decrease your risk of complications from a particular disease you already have, such as blindness resulting from diabetes?
- Is it to reduce the likelihood of having another heart attack?
- Is it to increase your energy level?

Motivational Scale

You may want to ask yourself another question regarding your commitment to this program. Rate yourself, with 10 being most confident or motivated.

Will I commit to this program?									
1	2	3	4	5	6	7	8	9	10

If you scored 7 or greater, your chance of success will be high. If you scored below 7, try to identify barriers that you believe will keep you from committing to the program. Then determine what it would take for you to rate yourself a 7 or greater. Could one of the barriers be that you've tried to lose weight and commit to an exercise program many times in the past and were unsuccessful? Or perhaps that you lost weight before but gained it back?

The Health First program is different. It is simple to follow, focuses on reducing your risk of getting many diseases, improves your sense of well-being, and provides you with a great deal more energy and vitality. The techniques for maintaining your weight loss are very practical. They have worked for many people. So join in, and be transformed!

Once you feel motivated to act and to take control of your health, the next step is to take some very simple baseline measurements. In my clinic, I use two simple tools: a tape measure and a scale. Weight and height measurements allow me to calculate a patient's body mass index (BMI), and the tape measure allows me to measure their waist circumference. These measurements help me determine their risk of disease. (I will collect other information that also helps determine risk. These include blood pressure, blood sugar, cholesterol, family history, and smoking history.)

Tomorrow morning, as soon as you get out of bed, fill in the following chart.

DATE

_____

HEIGHT

_____

WEIGHT

_____

WAIST CIRCUMFERENCE

_____

Calculating waist circumference.
While you're breathing out,
place the tape measure behind
your back and pull it around in a
level line to just a little above your
navel. Have someone help you if
you find this awkward.

Find Your BMI

Now you need to calculate your body mass index. There are
hundreds of BMI calculators on the Internet, but here is a useful
chart to help you put the number in context. (See also the Internet
site <www.diabetes.ca/bmi>.)

BMI values are categorized as: Underweight (<18.5), Healthy Weight (18.5 – 24.9), Overweight (25 – 29.9), Obese Class I (30 – 34.9), Obese Class II (35 – 39.9), Obese Class III (>40).

Stone	lbs	4'10" (147.3 cm)	4'11" (149.9 cms)	5'0" (152.4 cms)	5'1" (154.9 cms)	5'2" (157.5 cms)	5'3" (160.0 cms)	5'4" (162.6 cms)	5'5" (165.1 cms)	5'6" (167.6 cms)	5'7" (170.2 cms)	5'8" (172.7 cms)	5'9" (175.3 cms)	5'10" (177.8 cms)	5'11" (180.3 cms)	6'0" (182.9 cms)	6'1" (185.4 cms)	6'2" (188.0 cms)	6'3" (190.5 cms)	kgs
7st 2 lbs	100	20.9	20.2	19.6	18.9	18.3	17.8	17.2	16.7	16.2	15.7	15.2	14.8	14.4	14.0	13.6	13.2	12.9	12.5	45.5 kgs
7st 7lbs	105	22.0	21.3	20.5	19.9	19.2	18.6	18.1	17.5	17.0	16.5	16.0	15.5	15.1	14.7	14.3	13.9	13.5	13.2	47.7 kgs
7st 12 lbs	110	23.0	22.3	21.5	20.8	20.2	19.5	18.9	18.3	17.8	17.3	16.8	16.3	15.8	15.4	14.9	14.5	14.2	13.8	50.0 kgs
8 st 3 lbs	115	24.1	23.3	22.5	21.8	21.1	20.4	19.8	19.2	18.6	18.0	17.5	17.0	16.5	16.1	15.6	15.2	14.8	14.4	52.3 kgs
8 st 8 lbs	120	25.1	24.3	23.5	22.7	22.0	21.3	20.6	20.0	19.4	18.8	18.3	17.8	17.3	16.8	16.3	15.9	15.4	15.0	54.5 kgs
8st 13 lbs	125	26.2	25.3	24.5	23.7	22.9	22.2	21.5	20.8	20.2	19.6	19.0	18.4	18.0	17.5	17.0	16.5	16.1	15.7	56.8 kgs
9 st 4 lbs	130	27.2	26.3	25.4	24.6	23.8	23.1	22.4	21.7	21.0	20.4	19.8	19.2	18.7	18.2	17.7	17.2	16.7	16.3	59.1 kgs
9st 9 lbs	135	28.3	27.3	26.4	25.6	24.7	24.0	23.2	22.5	21.8	21.2	20.6	20.0	19.4	18.9	18.3	17.8	17.4	17.0	61.4 kgs
10 st 0 lbs	140	29.3	28.3	27.4	26.5	25.7	24.9	24.1	23.3	22.6	22.0	21.3	20.7	20.1	19.6	19.0	18.5	18.0	17.5	63.6 kgs
10 st 5 lbs	145	30.4	29.3	28.4	27.5	26.6	25.7	24.9	24.2	23.5	22.8	22.1	21.5	20.8	20.3	19.7	19.2	18.7	18.2	65.9 kgs
10 st 10 lbs	150	31.4	30.4	29.4	28.4	27.5	26.6	25.8	25.0	24.3	23.5	22.9	22.2	21.6	21.0	20.4	19.8	19.3	18.8	68.2 kgs
11st 1 lbs	155	32.5	31.4	30.3	29.3	28.4	27.5	26.7	25.8	25.1	24.3	23.6	22.9	22.3	21.7	21.1	20.5	19.9	19.4	70.5 kgs
11 st 6 lbs	160	33.5	32.4	31.3	30.3	29.3	28.4	27.5	26.7	25.9	25.1	24.4	23.7	23.0	22.4	21.7	21.2	20.6	20.0	72.7 kgs
11 st 11 lbs	165	34.6	33.4	32.3	31.2	30.2	29.3	28.4	27.5	26.7	25.9	25.1	24.4	23.7	23.1	22.4	21.8	21.2	20.7	75.0 kgs
12 st 2 lbs	170	35.6	34.4	33.3	32.2	31.2	30.2	29.2	28.4	27.5	26.7	25.9	25.2	24.4	23.8	23.1	22.5	21.9	21.3	77.3 kgs
12 st 7 lbs	175	36.7	35.4	34.2	33.1	32.1	31.1	30.1	29.2	28.3	27.5	26.7	25.9	25.2	24.5	23.8	23.1	22.5	21.9	79.5 kgs
12 st 12 lbs	180	37.7	36.4	35.2	34.1	33.0	32.0	31.0	30.0	29.1	28.3	27.4	26.6	25.9	25.2	24.5	23.8	23.2	22.5	81.8 kgs
13 st 3 lbs	185	38.7	37.4	36.2	35.0	33.9	32.8	31.8	30.8	29.9	29.0	28.2	27.4	26.6	25.9	25.1	24.5	23.8	23.2	84.1 kgs
13 st 8 lbs	190	39.8	38.5	37.2	36.0	34.8	33.7	32.7	31.7	30.7	29.8	28.9	28.1	27.3	26.6	25.8	25.1	24.4	23.8	86.4 kgs
13 st 13 lbs	195	40.8	39.5	38.2	36.9	35.7	34.6	33.5	32.5	31.5	30.6	29.7	28.9	28.0	27.3	26.5	25.8	25.1	24.4	88.6 kgs
14 st 4 lbs	200	41.9	40.5	39.1	37.9	36.7	35.5	34.4	33.4	32.3	31.4	30.5	29.6	28.8	28.0	27.2	26.4	25.7	25.1	90.9 kgs
14 st 9 lbs	205	42.9	41.5	40.1	38.8	37.6	36.4	35.3	34.2	33.2	32.2	31.2	30.3	29.5	28.7	27.9	27.1	26.4	25.7	93.2 kgs
15 st 0 lbs	210	44.0	42.5	41.1	39.8	38.5	37.3	36.1	35.0	34.0	33.0	32.0	31.3	30.2	29.4	28.5	27.8	27.0	26.3	95.5 kgs
15 st 5 lbs	215	45.0	43.5	42.1	40.7	39.4	38.2	37.0	35.9	34.8	33.7	32.8	31.8	30.9	30.0	29.2	28.4	27.7	26.9	97.7 kgs
15 st 10 lbs	220	46.1	44.5	43.1	41.7	40.3	39.1	37.8	36.7	35.6	34.5	33.5	32.6	31.6	30.7	29.9	29.1	28.3	27.6	100.0 kgs
16 st 1 lbs	225	47.1	45.5	44.0	42.6	41.2	39.9	38.7	37.5	36.4	35.3	34.3	33.3	32.4	31.4	30.6	29.7	28.9	28.2	102.3 kgs

Stone	lbs	4'10"	4'11"	5'0"	5'1"	5'2"	5'3"	5'4"	5'5"	5'6"	5'7"	5'8"	5'9"	5'10"	5'11"	6'0"	6'1"	6'2"	6'3"	kgs
16 st 6 lbs	230	48.2	46.6	45.0	43.5	42.2	40.8	39.6	38.4	37.2	36.1	35.0	34.0	33.1	32.1	31.3	30.4	29.6	28.8	104.5 kgs
16 st 11 lbs	235	49.2	47.6	46.0	44.5	43.1	41.7	40.4	39.2	38.0	36.9	35.8	34.8	33.8	32.8	31.9	31.1	30.2	29.4	106.8 kgs
17 st 2 lbs	240	50.3	48.6	47.0	45.4	44.0	42.6	41.3	40.0	38.8	37.7	36.6	35.5	34.5	33.5	32.6	31.7	30.9	30.1	109.1 kgs
17 st 7 lbs	245	51.3	49.6	47.9	46.4	44.9	43.5	42.1	40.9	39.6	38.5	37.3	36.3	35.2	34.2	33.3	32.4	31.5	30.7	111.4 kgs
17 st 12 lbs	250	52.4	50.6	48.9	47.3	45.8	44.4	43.0	41.7	40.4	39.2	38.1	37.0	35.9	34.9	34.0	33.1	32.2	31.3	113.6 kgs
18 st 3 lbs	255	53.4	51.6	49.9	48.3	46.7	45.3	43.9	42.5	41.2	40.0	38.9	37.7	36.7	35.6	34.7	33.7	32.8	31.9	115.9 kgs
18 st 8 lbs	260	54.5	52.6	50.9	49.2	47.7	46.2	44.7	43.4	42.1	40.8	39.6	38.5	37.4	36.3	35.3	34.4	33.5	32.6	118.2 kgs
18 st 13 lbs	265	55.5	53.6	51.9	50.2	48.6	47.0	45.6	44.2	42.9	41.6	40.4	39.2	38.1	37.0	36.0	35.0	34.1	33.2	120.5 kgs
19 st 4 lbs	270	56.5	54.6	52.8	51.2	49.5	47.9	46.4	45.0	43.7	42.4	41.1	40.0	38.8	37.7	36.7	35.7	34.7	33.8	122.7 kgs
19 st 9 lbs	275	57.6	55.7	53.8	52.1	50.4	48.8	47.3	45.9	44.5	43.2	41.9	40.7	39.5	38.4	37.4	36.4	35.4	34.4	125.0 kgs
20 st 0 lbs	280	58.6	56.7	54.8	53.0	51.3	49.7	48.2	46.7	45.3	43.9	42.7	41.4	40.3	39.1	38.1	37.0	36.0	35.1	127.3 kgs
20 st 5 lbs	285	59.7	57.7	55.8	54.0	52.2	50.6	49.0	47.5	46.1	44.7	43.4	42.2	41.0	39.8	38.7	37.7	36.7	35.7	129.5 kgs
20 st 10 lbs	290	60.7	58.7	56.8	54.9	53.2	51.5	49.9	48.4	46.9	45.5	44.2	42.9	41.7	40.5	39.4	38.3	37.3	36.3	131.8 kgs
21 st 1 lbs	295	61.8	59.7	57.7	55.9	54.1	52.4	50.7	49.2	47.7	46.3	44.9	43.7	42.4	41.2	40.1	39.0	38.0	36.9	134.1 kgs
21 st 6 lbs	300	62.8	60.7	58.7	56.8	55.0	53.3	51.6	50.0	48.5	47.1	45.7	44.4	43.1	41.9	40.8	39.7	38.6	37.6	136.4 kgs
21 st 11 lbs	305	63.9	61.7	59.7	57.7	55.9	54.1	52.5	50.9	49.3	47.9	46.5	45.1	43.9	42.6	41.5	40.3	39.2	38.2	138.6 kgs
22 st 2 lbs	310	64.9	62.7	60.7	58.7	56.8	55.0	53.3	51.7	50.1	48.7	47.2	45.9	44.6	43.3	42.1	41.0	39.9	38.8	140.9 kgs
22 st 7 lbs	315	66.0	63.8	61.6	59.6	57.7	55.9	54.2	52.5	50.9	49.4	48.0	46.6	45.3	44.0	42.8	41.6	40.5	39.5	143.2 kgs
22 st 12 lbs	320	67.0	64.8	62.6	60.6	58.7	56.8	55.0	53.4	51.8	50.2	48.8	47.4	46.0	44.7	43.5	42.3	41.2	40.1	145.5 kgs
23 st 3 lbs	325	68.1	65.8	63.6	61.5	59.6	57.7	55.9	54.2	52.6	51.0	49.5	48.1	46.7	45.4	44.2	43.0	41.8	40.7	147.7 kgs
23 st 8 lbs	330	69.1	66.8	64.6	62.5	60.5	58.6	56.8	55.0	53.4	51.9	50.3	48.8	47.4	46.1	44.8	43.6	42.5	41.3	150.0 kgs
23 st 13 lbs	335	70.2	67.8	65.6	63.4	61.4	59.5	57.6	55.9	54.2	52.6	51.0	49.6	48.2	46.8	45.5	44.3	43.1	42.0	152.3 kgs
24 st 4 lbs	340	71.2	68.8	66.5	64.4	62.3	60.4	58.5	56.7	55.0	53.4	51.8	50.3	48.9	47.5	46.2	45.0	43.7	42.6	154.5 kgs
24 st 9 lbs	345	72.3	69.8	67.5	65.3	63.2	61.2	59.3	57.5	55.8	54.1	52.6	51.1	49.6	48.2	46.9	45.6	44.4	43.2	156.8 kgs
25 st 0 lbs	350	73.3	70.8	68.5	66.3	64.1	62.1	60.2	58.4	56.6	54.9	53.3	51.8	50.3	48.9	47.6	46.3	45.0	43.8	159.1 kgs
25 st 5 lbs	355	74.4	71.9	69.5	67.2	65.1	63.0	61.1	59.2	57.4	55.7	54.1	52.5	51.0	49.6	48.2	46.9	45.7	44.5	161.4 kgs
cms		147.3 cm	149.9 cms	152.4 cms	154.9 cms	157.5 cms	160.0 cms	162.6 cms	165.1 cms	167.6 cms	170.2 cms	172.7 cms	175.3 cms	177.8 cms	180.3 cms	182.9 cms	185.4 cms	188.0 cms	190.5 cms	

Categories: Underweight <18.5 · Healthy Weight 18.5 - 24.9 · Overweight 25 - 29.9 · Obese Class I 30 - 34.9 · Obese Class II 35 - 39.9 · Obese Class III > 40

Using the BMI Chart

This BMI chart is designed so you can use units of measure with which you are most familiar – whether pounds, feet, and inches, or kilograms and centimeters. It is always best to have an accurate indication of your weight and height before finding your BMI. Following are illustrations of how to use the chart.

Example 1: Consider someone who weighs 200 pounds and is 5 feet, 8 inches tall. On the BMI chart, the pounds (lbs) are in a vertical column on the left, just to the right of the stones column. Horizontally, along the top of the chart, are the feet and inches. So, in this example, one would find 200 lbs almost halfway down along the vertical column on the left entitled lbs, and would find 5 feet, 8 inches (5' 8") along the horizontal line across the top of the chart. Follow along both lines to identify the point in the body of the BMI chart at which the two intersect. In this case, that point indicates a BMI of 30.5, which falls within Obese Class I or Category 1 Obesity.

Example 2: Consider someone who weighs 90.9 kilograms and is 57.5 centimeters in height. On the BMI chart, the kilograms (kg) are in the vertical column to the far right of the chart, and the centimeters (cm) are along a horizontal line at the bottom of the chart. Finding 90.5 kg along the right side of the chart, and 57.5 cm along the bottom, and following along both lines will bring you to the point in the body of the BMI chart where they intersect at a BMI reading of 36.7, which falls within Obese Class II or Category 2 Obesity.

Write down your BMI measurement and the date on which you calculated it. (Note that if you're of South Asian, Japanese, or Chinese descent, the BMI categories will have to be adjusted downward because of the generally smaller frame size of these populations.)

BMI _____

DATE _____

Now let's look at what this number means regarding your risk of common lifestyle diseases.

What BMI Means Regarding Your Risk of Disease					
Too thin	*Healthy category*	*Overweight category*	*Obesity category I*	*Obesity category II*	*Obesity category III*
BMI: less than 18.5	BMI: 18.5-24.9	BMI: 25-29.9	BMI: 30-34.9	BMI: 35-39.9	BMI: 40 or higher
	Healthy	Increased risk	High risk	Very high risk	Extremely high risk

Suppose your BMI falls in the healthy category or even a few numbers into the overweight category. If you have no other risk factors, I wouldn't be very concerned and would usually say, "See you next year." **If your BMI is 28 or higher, you most likely have a lifestyle health risk.**

Small Improvements Go a Long Way

Even if it takes you a long while to get out of the obesity category, just dropping 5% to 10% of your overall weight will significantly improve your risk profile and will make you feel better, too.

Waist Circumference and Disease Risk

Like most simple scales, BMI isn't perfect. Critics say it doesn't adequately account for people who are very muscular. It isn't fool-proof. The best predictor of disease risk is BMI combined with waist circumference.

It turns out that your belly is a reflection of what's going on inside your abdomen. Research shows that fat cells around internal organs, also known as visceral fat, seem to disrupt the normal hormonal balance in the body and are also associated with a higher risk of many diseases.

Tape Measures Are Not Just for Tailors

BMI isn't the only predictor of risk. With a BMI between 25 and 34.9, your risk becomes even more serious if you carry a lot of your weight around your waist. Within the BMI range of 25 and 34.9, there is a strong correlation between waist circumference and type 2 diabetes, coronary vascular disease, and high blood pressure.

How Disease Risk Increases with Waist Circumference in Certain BMI Ranges	
BMI	Waist circumference
	Men >40 inches (>102cm) Women >35 inches (>88cm) (present North American guide)
25-29.9	High risk
30-34.9	Very high risk
Source: <http://www.nhlbi.nih.gov/guidelines/obesity/e_txtbk/txgd/4142.htm> (1/6/12).	

The waist circumference danger zones presented above reflect guidelines provided by North American experts. These numbers are higher than those in guidelines published by European groups. Likewise, guidelines for people of South Asian, Chinese, and Japanese descent are lower. It's important to use the waist circumference guideline for your ethnicity, keeping in mind that guidelines change as our knowledge of disease risk continues to improve.

Waist Circumference Danger Zone		
* Europids (European descent) * Sub-Saharan Africans * Eastern Mediterranean and Middle Eastern populations	Male	≥ 37 inches (94cm)
	Female	≥ 31.5 inches (80cm)
* South Asians * Chinese * Ethnic South and Central Americans	Male	≥ 35.4 inches (90cm)
	Female	≥ 31.5 inches (80cm)
* Japanese	Currently undetermined. Use Asian values	
International Diabetes Federation in Europe Guidelines and Ethnicity <idf.org> (3/6/12).		

Understanding Your Cholesterol Numbers

It's widely known that it is generally best to have high HDL (good cholesterol) and low LDL (bad cholesterol) and triglycerides. Your physician can tell you what your ideal numbers should be, a determination made based on your ten-year cardiovascular risk score. Just remember that high LDL cholesterol is a significant risk factor for heart disease and stroke. These diseases also increase your risk of dementia.

Cholesterol numbers have a way of creeping up with increasing weight. It is important to be proactive and deal with cholesterol before you have a problem. I've always believed that it's far easier to prevent a problem than to correct one.

Record your most recent checkup results here:

DATE _____

LDL (bad cholesterol) _____

HDL (good cholesterol) _____

TRIGLYCERIDES _____

BLOOD PRESSURE _____ / _____

FASTING BLOOD SUGAR _____

What's Your Risk?

You Can't Change Your Family

What are your BMI, waist circumference, cholesterol numbers, blood sugars, and blood pressure telling you about your future health risk? Whatever your numbers reveal, your risk may be higher if you have a parent or sibling with a history of any of the following conditions: heart disease, diabetes, high blood pressure, or high cholesterol. Fortunately, genes don't necessarily determine your fate – your own health choices can help shape your future.

Chances are you have picked up this book because you want to lose weight, improve your health, and feel great. However, you may not have realized your risk profile for major life-changing diseases until now.

If you're concerned about your risk profile, the good news is:

- Even a moderate amount of physical activity and cardio exercise can improve your HDL (good) cholesterol, which will decrease your risk of heart disease
- The Health First program is a simple, never-go-hungry diet that can reduce your BMI and waist circumference, which together will reduce your risk of getting today's lifestyle diseases

The baseline data you just recorded are not just for future reference. They should also serve to inspire you to action. The firmer your commitment to the Health First program, the better your chances of living a healthier and longer life.

Some Statistical Truths

- 27% of Americans over sixty-five have diabetes (American Diabetes Association)
- 25% of Canadians have diabetes or pre-diabetes (Canadian Diabetes Association)
- 53% of those in the obesity category have an increased chance of thyroid cancer[*]
- 40% of endometrial and esophageal cancers are attributed to obesity[*]

··

Patient Story: Feeling Fabulous

Charles, a fifty-four-year-old, was diagnosed with type 2 diabetes. His fasting blood sugar was 7.8 (140.4 American units). His weight was 215 pounds (97.7kg). His BMI was 33 (class I obesity category), and his waist circumference was 42.5 inches (108cm). We discussed options for treatment of his type 2 diabetes, and he decided to attempt a lifestyle program instead of starting on medication. Charles totally embraced the Health First program and lost

---

[*] National Cancer Institute.

38 pounds (17kg) at a rate of about 2 pounds (1kg) per week. This was in 2006. He power walks for thirty minutes at least four times a week. At the time of writing, his weight is still off, his blood sugar is always in the target range, and he has no complications from his diabetes. Here's his take on all this:

I feel so great and have so much energy. I feel fabulous about controlling my diabetes through lifestyle without the use of medication. I have lived this way for the last six years. I will never go back to my old way of eating and not exercising. I'm just so focused on what I eat, always aware of portion size, and I read labels all the time. The program works.

2

Mindfulness:

· ·

Making Conscious Choices

Mindfulness means paying attention in a particular way:
on purpose, in the present moment, and non-judgmentally.

—*Jon Kabat-Zim,* Mindfulness for Beginners

The best, and most sustainable, action starts with the mind, not the body. That's why I devote this chapter to helping you use your mind in a way that will make the rest of my program more logical and actionable.

What does the word "diet" bring to your mind? Most likely ...

- Hunger
- Deprivation
- Fatigue
- Calories
- Dessert (none)
- Loneliness
- Alcohol (none)
- Punishment
- Exhaustion
- Embarrassment
- Failure
- Nuisance

Most of us feel we have neither the physical nor the mental energy to go on a strict diet, and we secretly resent the time it takes to think about food. We like to eat for pleasure as well as to satisfy our hunger. Having to plan our meals with forethought is punishment for most of us.

All these negative feelings jeopardize the likelihood that we will achieve permanent weight loss. It doesn't have to be that way. Let me introduce you to a new way of thinking about eating and dieting that shouldn't summon all these nasty associations. It hinges on being mindful, making healthy choices, and budgeting your portions as you do your money.

··

Patient Story: Feeling More Alive

Geoff is a sixty-nine-year-old who has had type 2 diabetes for the past twelve years. He needed to lose 50 to 60 pounds, as he was tired of carrying around so much weight and wanted to better control his diabetes with a lifestyle change. He hoped to decrease some of the medication he was on and didn't want to take insulin. "I just decided that I needed to take charge of my health," he says.

Geoff has now lost 46 pounds on the Health First program and has been able to stop one of his diabetes medications as his blood sugar is in much better control. As he puts it:

I feel so much more alive with all this weight off. I sleep so much better now, and I believe the cardio exercise that I'm doing four days a week has also helped my sleep. I like the concept of choosing healthy options instead of thinking about restricting what I can eat. The other day I had to carry something that weighed 40 pounds – I could not believe that I used to carry that much weight around all the time. I know I will reach my goal weight and keep it off. Choosing smaller portions, staying focused, being physically active daily, and exercising are the keys. I'm now much less fearful of developing kidney failure as a result of my diabetes, as my blood sugar is so much better since I have lost all this weight. This program really does work.

Mindfulness: Concentrate on What You're Eating

Eating is something we all have to do. We just do too much of it, often without even being aware of what we're doing. We scarcely notice the bowl of potato chips eaten while watching a movie. Or the bag of corn chips that vanishes in a few minutes.

Patients who have successfully lost weight on my program tell me that the single most important thing they learned was to be fully focused on what they were doing with food. They learned to focus on what they were eating, when they were eating, and why they were eating at a particular time. Being mindful of food, and your relationship to it, is an extremely valuable tool in losing weight.

Be mindful of what you're eating. Focus your attention on the portion you've taken, the health value of your selections, and the appropriateness of your choice in relation to your long-term health goals.

Bring your full attention to food whenever you're around it – whether you're preparing food, ordering food, opening the cupboard or fridge, going out for dinner, or visiting friends and family.

After a very short time, this mindfulness will become second nature to you. It isn't all that difficult. Those with peanut or shellfish allergies must be aware of food as a matter of life and death. For those who simply want to lose weight, what first seems like a task easily becomes second nature.

The more attention you pay to what you're eating, the healthier your choices become.

Q. You have a potentially fatal shellfish allergy. You're at a buffet. How will you eat?

A. **By focusing on every food choice.**

Most of us eat too quickly and without much thought as to what we're putting in our mouths. A critical component of the Health First program is learning to become focused on what you eat. When you pay more attention to your food, you'll eat less, make healthier choices, eat smaller portions, and lose weight.

There's no doubt that we're living in a society that contributes to becoming overweight or obese. Everywhere we turn, there is an abundance of easily available food poised to make us unhealthy and increase our risk of lifestyle diseases. For example, many of us have unhealthy foods in our cupboards, co-workers may bring sweets to share at work, convenience stores are filled with a huge variety of unhealthy snack foods, and fast food restaurants are busier than ever, serving foods high in saturated fats and sugars in portions that continue to grow. Food surrounds us, and rarely is convenient food good for us.

These trends may seem impossible to resist, but you are capable of fighting back, losing weight, and becoming healthier. Always think before you eat: Is there a healthier choice?

Think Before You Eat

Preventing mindless eating and staying focused around food will get you a long way toward reaching your weight-loss goals. Later, I'll provide you with some tips on managing at restaurants and social functions.

Contemporary Portions Are Gigantic

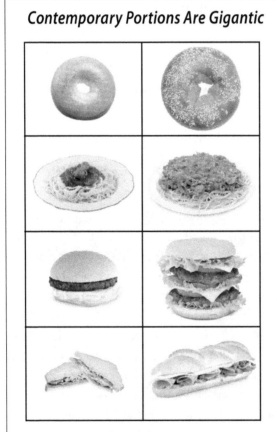

Portion creep is a major cause of obesity around the world. Food portions are double those common in the 1950s and, in some cases, even three times as large. You can see how the portion size on the left (1950s) compares to present day portion sizes on the right.

The National Heart, Lung, and Blood Institute has assembled these portion creep facts in a video called *Portion Distortion*.

Portion Size		
	Twenty Years Ago	**Today**
Bagel	3 inches	6 inches
Cheeseburger	333 calories	590 calories
Spaghetti	1 cup of pasta	2 cups of pasta
Fries	2.4 ounces	6.9 ounces
Turkey sandwich	320 calories	820 calories
Soda	7 fluid ounces	20 fluid ounces

Making Choices

I want you to think about food as something you have a choice about. Instead of feeling deprived of food because you're on a "diet," think of food as a tool to health and as something about which you always have a choice. You can choose a cookie, or you can choose an apple. You're not "giving up" the cookie. Instead, you're choosing to have a more wholesome snack that will advance your goal of having a healthy mind and body. You can have that cookie or saturated-fat-laden hamburger any time you want. You're simply choosing to make a healthier selection, one you won't regret the next time you have your cholesterol checked.

On the Health First program, you don't have to give up all that much of anything; you just budget your portions and make health-conscious selections. You'll gain empowerment over food by simply making better choices.

Tonight you may have a choice between cheesecake for dessert or fresh strawberries. You know the cheesecake is loaded with saturated fats and sugar, both of which will increase your risk of diabetes, heart disease, breast cancer, and colon cancer. Does this mean you can never have a piece of cheesecake again? Of course not. Once you reach your weight goal, you'll be able to choose a dessert once a week. It's also likely that you're not going to want to choose foods that are high in sugar and saturated fats very often. Your new "culture of health," as I call it, learned through a focus on mindfulness, will set you free from bad eating habits. (We'll talk more about this later, and how you can maintain your weight loss.)

Budgeting

Just as you budget your personal finances or your expense account, you can budget your portions of certain foods. Don't worry, there aren't many food groups to remember. I've made the Health First program very simple to follow. For each of the food groups, you'll be able to eat a certain number of portions per day or per week. Think of it as a budget that you can spend but not exceed. The details are explained in chapter 3; meanwhile, here's an example of what I mean.

For meats (beef, veal, lamb, and all pork products), you can have three portions per week. A meat portion is defined as 6 ounces (or 170 grams). As a rough guide, a 6-ounce meat portion (170 grams) is about the size of the palm of your hand. For example, you could have a 6-ounce steak on Monday night and have two portions left for the rest of the week. You could have 6 ounces of roast beef on Saturday night for dinner, and then have a 6-ounce lean burger on Sunday, and still be within your budget of three meat portions per week. The budget is three portions, any time during the week – but no more than 18 ounces (510 grams) of meat a week.

For many, this may be a real challenge; however, you may be comforted to know that poultry (chicken and turkey)* and vegetables are completely unlimited in this program. You are also allowed three fish portions per week. By following this simple program, you won't be hungry and you will feel great.

As you get further into the diet part of the program, don't forget to keep moving. Exercise and physical activity are every bit as important as diet for your overall health. (See chapter 7, "The Power of Moving.")

---

* Except if you have kidney disease.

Use Physical Activity as a Diversion

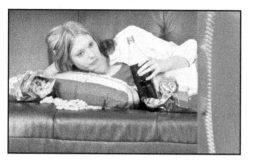

If you have a habit of eating while watching TV, try walking on a treadmill instead of snacking. Some of my patients now enjoy their shows this way. If you still want to snack while watching your favorite show, then choose a healthy snack like vegetables dipped in hummus, a piece of fruit, a handful of almonds or seeds, or plain yogurt (1% fat or less) with your own fresh fruit added to it.

Instead of eating mindlessly, try going for a walk, taking the dog out, throwing a ball with the kids, doing some yard work, or picking up the vacuum cleaner – anything active that will keep your hands busy, your mind distracted, and your body healthy.

Emotional Eating

Food is also tied to our emotions. Many of us eat in response to emotional states. Sometimes we eat out of boredom, depression, frustration, worry, disappointment, or anger. In my experience, for some patients, emotional eating is one of the biggest obstacles to overcome in trying to lose weight. Emotional eating often results in binging on unhealthy foods. Here are some techniques to try when the urge to comfort yourself with food comes upon you.

Be Mindful of Your Emotions

Recognize the emotion that's driving you to eat and confront it. Acknowledge it, give yourself permission to feel the way you do, but don't give yourself permission to let that negative emotion dictate bad eating habits. Don't use food to cope with emotions. Call a friend or do something to distract yourself from your emotional state. For those who snack on unhealthy foods out of boredom, or want to reward themselves for a hard day or a job well done, you could grab some baby carrots, cherry tomatoes, wedges of orange, red or yellow peppers, or a piece of fruit instead. These are much healthier choices, and they also taste great.

Be Prepared Inside and Outside the House

When it comes to food, preparation is almost as good as prevention. If you have a tendency toward emotional binge eating, make sure you always have lots of prepared vegetables in your refrigerator ready to eat. Keep some no-fat or 1% plain yogurt or hummus for dipping. Think of these as supplies that must be readily at hand. Without them, you're likely to turn to crackers, cookies, and other foods that are immediately available but will not help you reach your goals.

Plan to take a healthy snack with you whenever you're going to work or when you're shopping or going to a movie.

A Trick That Always Works

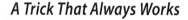

On your way home from work or on your way to a restaurant, eat a piece of fruit or a small container of plain yogurt or handful of almonds. Fruit or yogurt consumed twenty minutes to a half hour before you eat will cut your appetite. Taking the edge off your hunger will make you far less likely to grab the first thing that comes to hand at home or to overeat at a restaurant.

No fruit or yogurt with you? A bottle of water fifteen minutes before a meal will also moderate your hunger.

A New Meaning to "Bring Your Own"

Do big family meals create a huge temptation to splurge? One of my patients participating in the Health First program made a point of bringing a plate of cut-up vegetables and fruit to family gatherings so she could enjoy healthy snacking before and after the big meal. (She has lost 29 pounds and has kept them off.)

Creating mindfulness by following these simple steps will provide you with insights into your eating behaviors. This is the first important step to achieving a healthy lifestyle.

Patient Story: Feeling Great – and Safe

Mary is a fifty-eight-year-old with a BMI of 34 and a waist circumference of 38.6 inches (98cm). She was pre-diabetic. A year later, she was diagnosed with colon cancer. After her surgery, she was determined to lose weight to avoid developing diabetes and to help reduce her risk for a recurrence of colon cancer.

She embraced the Health First program and lost 20 pounds (10kg) over three months. Her blood sugar is now normal and, to date, her colon cancer has not returned. As she writes:

I feel great and I'm so proud of myself. So many of my friends in our community have type 2 diabetes, and I now feel totally confident that I have prevented getting it myself by losing 20 pounds and making exercise part of my lifestyle. I also feel very strongly that my new way of living will prevent my colon cancer from coming back.

3

The Key to Success:

. . . .

The Diet That Satisfies and Works

What you get by achieving your goals
is not as important as what you become
by achieving your goals.

—Goethe

The Health First program is as effective as it is simple. By choosing healthier foods, controlling your portion sizes, and budgeting your food groups, you'll lose weight. Not only that, but you'll learn to change your eating habits permanently and keep the weight off forever.

During the Active Weight Loss part of the overall program, desserts will be off limits other than fruit that is within your allotted budget.

You'll be encouraged to seek out whole grains and a large variety of vegetables and fruit. You will also learn to eat less red meat but more fish and poultry. By reducing the saturated fats found in rich desserts, red meat, cheese, and high-fat dairy products, your risk of developing colon cancer, breast cancer, and heart disease will be significantly reduced. And you'll lose weight, too.

During the Weight Maintenance part of the program, while continuing to closely monitor your food group choices, you'll be able to add some starch choices and treat yourself to occasional desserts.

As I've seen with my patients, budgeting portions will give you more control over your food choices, give you lots of flexibility, and prevent you from feeling deprived and hungry.

This chapter takes an in-depth look at all the different food groups. I define how much of these foods you may eat in a period of a week. Then, in the next chapter, I suggest daily meal plans incorporating the items from these food groups.

Just one caveat. Don't let yourself get hungry. **Hunger wins every time.** Skipping meals is never a good idea. Breakfast is critical in managing your appetite, your energy, and your ability to think and learn. It is very important to have three solid meals every day. Throughout the rest of the day, enjoy three or four healthy snacks and drink lots of water. Learn to enjoy a variety of fruit and vegetables.

Don't let yourself get hungry. Hunger always wins. Never skip meals. Stay mindful of what you're eating at all times.

Patient Story: A New Lease on Life

To get you motivated, consider Frank, a sixty-eight-year-old who had a BMI of 36 (class II obesity category) and a waist circumference of 45 inches (110cm). He had elevated blood pressure and cholesterol. Consequently, he was at great risk of heart attack, stroke, type 2 diabetes, and several cancers. My approach could have been to start him on blood pressure and cholesterol medication while advising him to lose weight and exercise. After a good discussion about his options for treatment and risk reduction, he agreed to follow the Health First program for weight loss and disease prevention, with me as his health coach. He chose not to start medication at this time.

By following the program, Frank lost 82 pounds (37kg). Both his blood pressure and cholesterol are perfectly normal now. He says he "loves doing exercise" and that it has become part of his life. "I have so much more energy. I feel like I'm in my twenties again. I have a new lease on life."

Frank successfully changed his lifestyle and dramatically changed his health profile. He significantly reduced his risk of developing osteoarthritis, type 2 diabetes, various cancers, heart disease, and stroke. (His wife lost 100 pounds on the Health First program as well, and she and Frank feel like a young couple again.)

Health First Food Groups

The food groups in this Health First program don't line up perfectly with the conventional ones you may have read about in other nutrition information. For example, some other programs include carbohydrates as a food group; however, carbohydrates include starches, vegetables, and fruit. Because starches are generally the component of this grouping that gets people into trouble, I prefer to break carbohydrates into three sub-groups: starches, vegetables, and fruit.

The following food groups are simple and give rise to an easy-to-follow plan for successful weight loss and better health.

Starches: cereal, bread, pasta, rice, potatoes, crackers, couscous, quinoa
Meat: beef, veal, lamb, all pork products
Poultry: chicken, turkey, duck
Fish: fish, shellfish
Vegetables
Fruit
Dairy: yogurt, milk
Cheese
Eggs
Legumes: beans, peas, lentils

Keep it simple. It works!
So let's get started. I will describe each of the food groups and indicate easy-to-measure portion sizes and a "budget" for each food group.

Starches

Cereal, bread, pasta, rice, potatoes, crackers, couscous, quinoa
• Must be whole grain, or whole wheat, or brown rice. No white bread, white flour, or white rice
• *1 portion = the size of your palm*
• *3 portions* **per day (females)**
• *4 portions* **per day (males)**
• Choose 100% whole grains

The Health First program begins with starches because starches – breads, cereals, pasta, rice, potatoes, and crackers – constitute the food group most likely to be enjoyed to excess.

Starch portions have become massive. Bagels and bread slices are larger today than they were fifty to sixty years ago. Pasta servings have grown tremendously, too. What we consider a normal portion today would have been at least two servings in the 1950s.

Portion creep is slowly killing us!

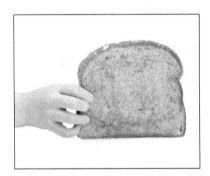 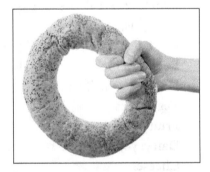

It is critical that, in addition to reducing the number and size of starch portions, you seek out whole grains.

Studies have shown that people who eat whole grains rather than refined grains (white bread, white rice, or regular pasta) have a lower risk of heart disease, obesity, and certain cancers. Always choose whole grain bread, whole grain cereal, whole wheat pasta, and brown or wild rice.

Whole grains not only are more nutritious but also have the benefit of not triggering insulin spikes after eating. When insulin goes up, blood sugar goes down and we feel hungry. This is why you typically feel satisfied longer after a meal with whole grains than after one with refined grains. It's a win/win.

Naturally, you'll want to avoid anything fried or fatty, which means passing on fries or creamy mashed potatoes. Remember – the food you eat is a choice, and you're choosing to be healthy. This isn't deprivation; it's innovation. There's a new, more vigorous you developing with each better choice you make.

Cereal

Whole grain only
• 1 portion = palm size (about ½ cup)
• HINT: Add real fruit to sweeten the cereal naturally.
• WARNING: Read cereal box labels. Select cereal brands that are low in sugar. (See chapter 5 for much more about sugars.)

Bread

Whole grain only
• 1 portion = palm size
• CAUTION: A standard slice of bread is 4 inches by 4.5 inches by ½ inch thick (10cm x 11cm x 2cm). Many slices these days are almost double this size.

Some of my patients think that, if they choose whole grain bread, they can eat as much as they want. This is not correct. Even whole grain bread must be counted as part of the budgeted starch portion for the day.

Watch the size of your bread portions, too. Many buns, bagels and slices of bread are altogether too large – double or triple what they used to be. Often a single slice of bread of a restaurant sandwich will fill your entire hand from your wrist to the tips of your fingers; it is equal to two slices, making the whole sandwich equivalent to four bread portions.

For a male, the restaurant-sized sandwich noted above would include a full day's budget of starch. For a female, the same sandwich would contain one starch portion in excess of the allowed budget. The solution would be to leave some of the bread uneaten, or choose a salad with tuna or grilled chicken instead. Try going to restaurants at lunchtime less often. It's always better to bring your own lunch so you can control your portions.

Treat your portion allowance like a budget. Once you've eaten your allowance, you can't have more. Overdrafts are not allowed.

Pasta

• *Whole wheat pasta only*
• *1 portion = palm size, about ½ cup*

Pasta dishes are the prime example of portion creep. The amount of pasta always fills the plate, and plates are getting larger. You must focus on portion size when eating pasta. Remember that one palm is one portion. Three starch portions equal approximately 1½ cups of pasta. If you have a starch for breakfast or lunch, a restaurant pasta dish will likely push you seriously over budget. When you plan to have pasta, add many cooked vegetables to the dish so your plate is full and you feel satisfied at the end of your meal.

Rice

• *Brown or wild rice only*
• *1 portion = palm size, about ½ cup*

As with bread and pasta, portion control is critical. Years ago, chicken or fish would be served on a slender bed of rice. Many restaurants today cover the plate with rice.

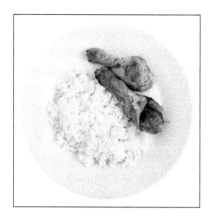 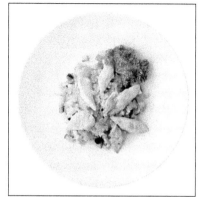

Even if you switch from white rice to healthier brown or wild rice, you must still stay within your starch budget. Healthy starches are still starches. Three servings for women and four servings for men is the budget per day.

Sample Budgeting for Starch Portions	
Breakfast	Half cup of cereal with 1% milk and some strawberries (1 starch portion)
Lunch	Grilled teriyaki salmon, 6oz Grilled vegetables and a salad
Dinner	Skinless chicken breast, grilled 1 cup of brown rice (2 starch portions) Generous portion of cooked vegetables and salad
	(You have 0 or 1 starch portions remaining, depending on whether you are female or male)

In this sample menu, a woman would have used up her starch budget for a day, whereas a man would have one starch portion left for a larger serving of rice or for a snack.

Potatoes

• Enjoy white or sweet potatoes
• **1 portion = palm size**

Potatoes come in all sizes. One portion fills the palm of your hand. You need to keep this in mind if you've baked a larger potato. Cut it in half to make sure you're not exceeding your budget. A handful of little potatoes would be one portion. A little butter is fine, but do without sour cream and bacon bits, both of which are full of saturated fat.

As for mashed potatoes, use discretion. Restaurants make them high in saturated fats by adding large amounts of butter, cream, and sometimes sour cream. If you make your own, use just a little butter and either 1% milk or plain low-fat yogurt. And remember: One portion equals the size of your palm.

Crackers

• *Whole wheat, watch portion size*
• *1 portion = palm size*

Couscous

• *Whole wheat*
• *1 portion = palm size, about ½ cup*

Quinoa

• *Gluten-free*
• *1 portion = palm size, about ½ cup*

Meat

Beef, veal, lamb, and pork products
• **3 portions of meat per week**
• **1 portion = 6oz (170g)**
• Avoid all processed meats such as sausage, bacon, smoked meat, corned beef, ham, pepperoni, salami, bologna, hot dogs, and processed chicken or turkey

People eating a typical Western-style diet consume too much red meat. Red meat significantly increases the risk of stroke, heart disease, breast cancer, colon cancer, and prostate cancer. The Health First program restricts the amount of meat you can eat to three 6-ounce (170g) portions per week.

If you're used to eating a lot of red meat, this restriction may be a small sacrifice. But chicken, turkey, and fish can be equally satisfying and are healthier choices.

Apart from paying attention to the size and frequency of your meat portions, you must also avoid processed meats such as bacon, sausage, ham, smoked meats, corned beef, and all cold cuts including processed chicken and turkey. Processed meats are loaded with saturated fats, nitrates, and sodium, all of which are very unhealthy.

Do not exceed your meat budget. Start keeping track of your meat consumption on Monday morning. Once you reach three meat portions, remind yourself daily that your meat budget is used up until the following Monday.

Red meat (beyond 18oz, or 510g per week) significantly increases the risk of getting heart disease, breast cancer, colon cancer, and prostate cancer.

Poultry

Chicken, turkey, duck, and Cornish hen
• **Unlimited portions of unprocessed, skinless chicken and turkey** per week
• *6oz (170g) of duck or Cornish hen per week*
• *Favor white meat over dark, always skinless*
• *Avoid fried and processed poultry*

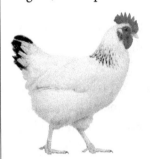 Baked, broiled, or roasted chicken and turkey, stripped of skin and fat, are wholesome and delicious. White meat has less fat than dark meat, so you should choose it more often. Again, avoid processed poultry that comes in a giant roll, or turkey infused with butter to increase tenderness. Eat the real thing. Avoid fried and processed chicken or turkey.

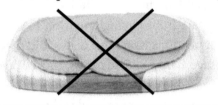

The Health First program allows you to have as many servings of poultry per week as you like. It's better for you to have an extra piece of chicken at a meal if you're hungry than to fill up with extra starches or junk food later in the evening. No one I know is overweight as a result of eating too much chicken (unless they're eating it fried).

If you have kidney disease, check with your doctor to discuss how much protein is safe for you.

Once a week, you may choose duck or Cornish hen. Always remember to take off the skin, as this contains a lot of saturated fat. With either duck or Cornish hen, limit yourself to six ounces (170gm) once a week.

Be careful of sauces. Ideally you should avoid sauces altogether, but non-fat sauces such as teriyaki or salsa can liven up a meal. Just watch for excess salt and sugar in sauces you select.

Fish

Fish and shellfish
• **3 portions** per week
• **1 portion = 6oz (170g)**
• Favor oily fish, but seek variety
• Avoid fried fish
• Shellfish may be one of 3 fish portions per week

Fish is certainly good for your heart. However, it should be eaten in moderation because of mercury concerns. Shellfish, too, needs to be treated with caution because it is generally high in cholesterol.

Omega-3 Fatty Acids

The fatty fishes are the preferred fishes because they are rich in omega-3 fatty acids, which is essential for cardiovascular health. The cold-water oily fishes are salmon, trout, tuna, herring, mackerel, and sardines. Following is a list of oily fishes.

Type of fish	Total omega-3 content per 3.5oz in grams
Mackerel	2.6
Trout (lake)	2.0
Herring	1.7
Tuna (bluefin)	1.6
Salmon	1.5
Sardines	1.5
Sturgeon	1.5
Tuna (albacore)	1.5
Whitefish (lake)	1.5
Anchovies	1.4
Bass (striped)	0.8
Trout (brook)	0.6
Trout (rainbow)	0.6

While you're on your weight-reduction program, fish and chips are out because they are fried foods. It's important for you, when you're in a restaurant, to avoid cream and butter-based sauces and to remember your portion size. Six ounces at one meal is the limit, three times a week.

I recommend restricting yourself to just one serving of shellfish per week in place of one of the fish selections. A note of warning here: if you have high cholesterol, heart disease, or have had a stroke, check with your doctor about the advisability of eating shellfish weekly.

About Mercury

The higher a particular fish is on the food chain, the more mercury it accumulates in its body. Larger fish such as swordfish and shark have higher concentrations of mercury than smaller fish such as salmon, herring, and shellfish.

Many people consume a lot of tuna. You should be aware that albacore canned tuna has more mercury than canned light tuna.

Tuna, salmon, or crab salad made with mayonnaise should be avoided while you're trying to lose weight. Try mixing canned fish with a small amount of calorie-reduced salad dressing or plain balsamic vinegar instead. Canned salmon works well with honey-flavored or horseradish mustard.

Vegetables

Unlimited – as much as you can eat
Seek variety
Prepare in advance
Potatoes are not included

Eating vegetables each and every day will reduce your risk of developing heart disease and cancer.

"There is strong research to show that eating a variety of vegetables can boost your health, and among other things, helps to reduce the risk of heart disease and cancer. Vegetables of all colors are a nutritional goldmine. The deeply colored ones are bursting with antioxidants that fight harmful compounds in our bodies" <www.Eatrightontario.ca>.

The Health First program considers all vegetables free and unlimited. (This does not include potatoes; nor does it include legumes, which are covered later in this chapter.) Eat as many vegetables as you would like, all day, every day, with all your meals, as snacks, and as a way to deal with hunger. Variety is key to nutritional balance and maximum benefit.

Try new varieties like collard, bok choy, leeks, Swiss chard, Belgium endive, fennel, and squash. Eat plenty of salad greens such as romaine lettuce, arugula, baby spinach, and spring mix. Try to eat as many different colors of vegetables as you can. The different colors all provide health-enhancing effects.

The Colorful World of Vegetables						
Greens	**Greens**	**Greens**	**Yellows**	**Reds**	**Purples**	**Whites**
Arugula	Cucumber	Peas	Yellow peppers	Tomatoes	Eggplant	Cauliflower
Asparagus	Endive	Rapini	Yellow tomatoes	Radishes	Purple cabbage	Turnip
Bok choy	Fennel	Snow peas	Carrots	Radicchio	Purple endive	Mushrooms
Broccoli	Green beans	Spinach	Pumpkin	Beets	Purple peppers	Onion
Brussels sprouts	Green lettuces	Swiss chard	Yellow summer squash	Red onion		Parsnip
Cabbage	Green pepper	Watercress	Butternut squash			Jicama
Celery	Kale	Zucchini	Winter squash			
Chinese cabbage	Leeks		Acorn squash			
Collard greens	Okra					

Cooking and Preparation

Steam or grill your vegetables. Even stir-frying is okay, so long as you use a heart-healthy oil, such as olive oil, somewhat sparingly. Speaking of oil, free your salads from smothering salad dressings – they are often high in sugar and the wrong kind of fat. It is best to use a light vinaigrette with an olive oil base to let the flavor come alive.

To be successful with vegetables, you should have lots of them in your refrigerator, and, ideally, they should be prepared in advance. Here is one approach: after dinner, gather some vegetables to prepare for that evening's snack and for the next day. Wash, peel, cut, portion, and store them in plastic storage bags and/or plastic re-sealable containers. This way you'll have some bags of vegetables to grab as you rush out of the house the next morning, as well as snacks should the urge hit you in the evening. If you don't eat them all, you're that much farther ahead in meal preparation for the next day, as you can likely use them in a stir-fry.

What About Corn and Carrots?

Patients with previous dieting experience sometimes ask if they should avoid corn, because of its starch, or carrots, because of their sugar content. Over many years of treating my patients with this successful program, no one has had difficulty losing weight or maintaining it because they ate too many carrots or too much corn. Just don't overdo it on corn.

In the Health First program, you can and should eat as many vegetables as you want, with a focus on having many different types of vegetables daily. Variety is indeed the spice of life – even with vegetables.

If you have already eaten your allotted starch budget, you should add an extra vegetable at subsequent meals to ensure that you feel satisfied. Let's say you had a sandwich at lunch. For dinner you could have a large piece of chicken breast, two different kinds of cooked vegetables, asparagus and broccoli for instance, and a large salad. That would constitute a full, satisfying meal.

Fruit

Fiber, Vitamins, and Antioxidants
• **4 portions per day**
• Eat fresh or frozen
• Seek out a wide variety
• **1 portion = palm size**
• Avoid fruit juices
• No added syrup, sugar, or sweeteners
• Use fruit strategically

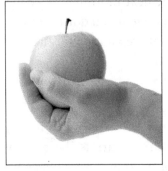 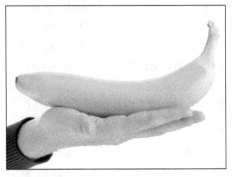

1 fruit portion   *2 fruit portions*

An apple a day may not truly keep the doctor away, but it's a good start. Fruits are full of vitamins and minerals. The Health First program requires four fruit portions a day – every day.

Why only four a day? Many people make the mistake of thinking that, because fruits are wholesome, an unlimited amount of them is a good thing. This is not correct. Several of my patients have developed pre-diabetes with no apparent cause other than excessive fruit consumption. Fruit contains a lot of natural sugars, which, if consumed in significant excess, can cause your blood sugar to rise, eventually leading to pre-diabetes. When these patients reduced their fruit consumption to four portions per day, their blood sugar returned to normal.

In addition to limiting how many fruits you can eat in one day, you must control the portion size of your fruit selections. Your palm is your measuring cup. If it fits in your palm, you've got a portion. A large banana that sticks out over both sides of your palm will likely be two portions. A grapefruit will typically be two portions. This is a rough guide, but it works well. Be careful with portion creep for other fruits as well; for example, think about how big some apples have recently become.

Eat a variety of different fruits and try to have them raw to maximize nutrients and fiber. Frozen or canned fruit is fine so long as it's not in sugary syrups. At the grocery store, explore fresh fruits that are new to you, including those from both tropical and temperate climates. Try to keep it interesting with seasonal fruit from all over the world. Support local growers, if you can, by going to your local farmers' market for your weekly fruit supply. Enjoy berries, melons, exotic fruits from the tropics or Asia, juicy peaches, ripe plums, nectarines, kiwi, passion fruit, and pears.

Apple	Pineapple	Grapes	Papaya	Cantaloupe
Blueberries	Orange	Grapefruit*	Peach	Fig
Honeydew	Raspberries	Pear	Plum	Kiwi
Apricot	Strawberries	Banana	Nectarine	Mango
Watermelon	Blackberries			
*If you're on medication, check with your doctor or pharmacist for possible interaction with grapefruit.				

About Juice

Enjoy fruit in its natural form, but avoid juices. Juice concentrates your fruit servings and will undermine your diet. Think of it: an 8-ounce glass of orange juice contains at least four to six squeezed oranges. Just one glass of juice will give you more than your daily fruit allotment. Not only that, but juice deprives you of much of the beneficial fiber of whole fruit as well as the chance to use fruit as a snack throughout the day.

Use Fruit Strategically

Fruit will help you manage your appetite and keep up your energy throughout the day. I suggest having a fruit mid-morning, another mid-afternoon, and one about a half hour before dinner. This will prevent you from feeling "starved," a feeling that invariably leads to overeating at mealtime and potentially to poor food choices. (Don't forget to drink lots of water, too.)

To make this strategy work, it helps to have fruit readily available at home, at work, in your car, purse, briefcase, or backpack. (This is also true of the other snacks this program encourages you to eat throughout the day.) If it isn't easy to grab, fruit is unlikely to be the food of choice. Be sure to have four pieces of fruit every day. You might consider putting fruit in your yogurt or on your cereal at breakfast, or one piece cut up into small pieces in the evening as a snack, to total no more than four portions a day.

The best and most pleasant way to manage your appetite is to use fruit to dampen your hunger before a meal. Other snacks throughout the day are useful and should be enjoyed as well. It is so important not to allow yourself to become hungry.

About Dried Fruit

Dried fruit is better than no fruit, but fresh or frozen fruit is best. It's too easy to exceed your daily fruit portion when you tear open a fresh bag of dried apricots or moist prunes. Keep in mind that one dried fruit portion counts as a fruit portion. Reading the nutrition facts on the back of the package will be very informative and will allow you to avoid packaged dried fruit that has added sugars.

Always remember that 1 portion of dried fruit = palm size.

Milk, Yogurt, and Milk Alternatives

3 portions per day
1 portion of milk = 1 cup
1 portion of yogurt = ¾ cup
Yogurt, plain, 1% or 0% fat
Milk, 1% or 0% fat
Substitute soy or almond milk, as desired

Like milk, yogurt is an excellent source of protein, but dairy products are generally very high in saturated fats. Adults should choose low-fat or zero-fat dairy products. It is so much healthier for you to drink 1% or skim milk and eat yogurt that is 1% or 0% fat rather than the higher-fat alternatives. The reason *plain yogurt* is so important is that the yogurt sold with added fruit is mainly sugar.

For example, a popular low-fat yogurt cup with added fruit sold at a coffee chain has 18 grams of sugar. This equates to 4.5 teaspoons of sugar.

I highly recommend that you buy plain, 0%, or 1% yogurt and add your own handful of fruit for flavor.

Plain yogurt is ideal for a snack. If you're not keen on its slightly sour taste, mix some fresh fruit and/or almonds into it, or sprinkle some cinnamon on it. You may think you're doing yourself a favor when you opt for yogurt with fruit already added, but these products are usually made with syrup, jelly, and/or artificial sweeteners. (More on this in chapter 5, on sugar.)

Choose Low or Zero-fat Dairy Products

You might explore soymilk and almond milk for nutritional variety and, for those with a lactose intolerance, as an alternative to milk.

Your three daily dairy portions can be any mix of milk, yogurt, and alternatives. Also, remember to count the milk you put in your coffee or tea, or in your cereal. Similarly, on days when you have cheese, you'll need to remember to cut your milk and milk alternatives down to just two portions.

Cheese – Use Caution

• *3 portions* per week
• *1 portion = 1.5oz (42.5g)*
• *If choosing low-fat cheese, be cautious*
• *Count cheese included in other dishes*

Although we have all grown up thinking that cheese is a healthy food, cheese is very high in saturated fats. While some weight-loss programs call for no dairy products at all, the Health First program allows you to have cheese, but limited to three portions per week. Exercise caution with low-fat cheese.

Don't be tempted to eat much more than an allowable portion just because it is low fat.

Be conscientious in keeping track of how much cheese you're eating, as it is extremely easy to exceed your weekly limit. Cheese is often added to sandwiches, pasta, and salads, where even small amounts can add up quickly. Always include in your weekly count the cheese in cheeseburgers, subs, quiches, and omelets, and on pizzas, and anything au gratin or with cream cheese. As with meat, you must remind yourself every day of your remaining weekly cheese budget allowance.

Remember, a day with a full cheese portion should be a day with one fewer milk and milk alternative.

Eggs – Any Way You Like 'em!

• 4 whole eggs per week
• Count eggs in dishes and baked goods

Eggs are a great source of protein. They also contain cholesterol, which is why we were urged for years to significantly limit our consumption of them. However, after many years of studies, it has been found that saturated fats, not cholesterol, are the main culprit in elevating our blood cholesterol.

So the bottom line on eggs? With the Health First program, you can safely have four whole eggs per week. However, if you already have high cholesterol, high blood pressure, or heart disease, check with your doctor first before following this recommendation.

At home, prepare eggs any way you like, but be mindful of added fat. When frying, use just a tiny amount of heart-healthy oil. Avoid egg salad with lots of mayonnaise, which is often the way it is served in restaurants. If you must have mayonnaise, choose the low-fat kind and use it sparingly. Remember that baked goods contain eggs, as do custards and many cream dishes. You should be avoiding these saturated fatty foods while you're trying to lose weight. Keep in mind that these foods often contain lots of sugar as well.

One other word of caution: Restaurant omelets can be made

with four eggs, which is your whole week's portion of eggs! When ordering an omelet at a restaurant, specify how many eggs you wish it to be made from and ask to have the cooking oil used sparingly. While you're at it, ask to have it without cheese and ask for extra sautéed vegetables instead.

Legumes

Beans, peas, lentils, soybeans
• *Up to 1 cup* per day
• *Eat a variety*

One cup of lentils, beans, peas, or tofu provides a rich source of fiber and protein. Although legumes are good for you, the Health First program limits them to just one cup a day. Some suggested legumes:

- Adzuki beans (red oriental beans)
- Anasazi beans (Jacob's cattle beans)
- Black beans (turtle beans)
- Black-eyed peas (cow peas)
- Chickpeas (garbanzo beans): the basis of hummus
- Edamame (green soybeans)
- Fava beans (horse beans)
- Lentils
- Lima beans (butter beans)
- Red kidney beans
- Soy nuts (roasted soybeans) – watch for excessive salt
- Sugar snap peas

Buy local for maximum freshness and environmental benefit.

Snacks

Healthy Snacking – 4 times a day!
• Make a habit of snacking on "tons" of vegetables
• Fruit is a great snack (but only 4 portions per day)
• Have a daily handful-sized portion of nuts and olives
• Eat a handful of seeds daily
• Use one of your 3 weekly cheese portions as a snack
• For best results, prepare your snacks in advance
• Always have a snack with you

Snacking is key to feeling satisfied, keeping up your energy level, and preventing feelings of deprivation. By snacks, I do not mean the common junk we pop in our mouths because it's available – like chips and candy bars, or even granola bars. The snacks you should be enjoying are vegetables, fruit, yogurt, hummus for dip, nuts, seeds, and occasionally some cheese (as long as it's within your weekly cheese budget). Your snacks have to be as healthy for you as the rest of your diet.

Planning your snacks will help you ensure that they're varied, interesting, and delicious. One trick is to pre-portion sandwich bags of fresh vegetables, pieces of fruit, occasional chunks of cheese, or assorted berries. You might consider packing a cooler bag with some yogurt or milk. Preparing your own trail mix with assorted nuts and seeds is also very helpful. Here are some great ideas that my patients have found helpful: try preparing carrots and celery with a hummus dip, mixing yogurt with cut-up fruit, and portioning some cheese and olives. Preplanning is an advantageous way to keep yourself on track with the program.

The joy of snacking is limited only by your imagination and preparation time. Just be cautious about portions. Of all the snacking options, only vegetables are unlimited – so eat lots of them.

Going to a restaurant, a party, or a function with lots of food?

I highly recommend having a snack half an hour ahead so you don't find yourself arriving there feeling starved. Should you find yourself en route to dinner without a snack, stop to buy a piece of fruit or some nuts or other beneficial snack. Snacking will be critical to your success in achieving your weight goals.

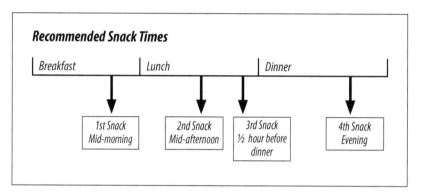

I recommend a mid-morning snack, a mid-afternoon snack, a mandatory snack half an hour before dinner, and an evening snack if necessary. Fruit is highly recommended for the mid-afternoon and pre-dinner snacks.

Nuts are a valuable source of omega-3 fats and fiber. You should eat a small handful of almonds, walnuts, or pecans every day. Peanuts are a good snack, too, but are not recommended every day and should be portioned when they are in the shell. Beware of commercial peanut butter, as it is higher in saturated fat than peanut butter from a health food store. It's best for you to limit your peanut butter to one tablespoon per week.

Seeds should be limited to a handful per day. Also, a handful of popcorn seeds are a good portion for an air popper, which is the recommended method for preparing popcorn. Add a light sprinkling of olive oil after popping. Sunflower, flax, and poppy seeds are all rich in important minerals and high in fiber.

Olives are another nutritious snack food, loaded with healthy oil and minerals. Eating a variety of colors and kinds is very healthy, but do your best to avoid those in brine, to keep your sodium intake down.

TV Watching

For those who must have something to eat while watching
your favorite show, you can prepare an assortment of raw
vegetables and some hummus for dipping. Having a glass
of cold sparkling water with lemon is also a great way to
consume a healthy drink. Having a small bowl of air-popped
popcorn is also allowable. Mindless eating at night can easily
jeopardize your success,
so stay focused and
be very mindful
about what
you're eating
and pre-portion
anything other
than vegetables.

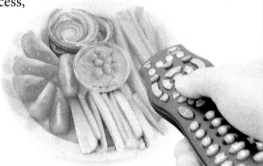

Snack Ideas: Be Creative

- Red, yellow, and orange peppers
- Broccoli florets
- Cherry tomatoes
- Almonds, walnuts, pecans
- Baby carrots
- Berries
- Air-popped popcorn
- Salsa dip for vegetables
- Your own trail mix
- Fruit cut into small pieces
- Carrot and celery sticks
- Dried fruit (handful)
- Bean salad with calorie-reduced dressing
- Yogurt (plain, 0% to 1% fat)
- Salad with calorie-reduced dressing
- Hummus for dipping vegetables

Alcohol

Alcohol, Yes, but Not Too Much
• **Females: Up to 4 drinks per week**
• **Males: Up to 7 drinks per week**

• **1 drink**
    = 1.5oz of liquor
    = 12oz of beer
    = 5oz of wine

Unlike many other diets, some alcohol is allowed. While on the Active Weight Loss part of the Health First program, men can have up to seven drinks per week and women up to four drinks per week. To keep on track with your weight-loss goals, remember not to mix fruit juices with alcohol, and definitely stay away from cocktails with syrups, mixes, or soft drinks.

In my experience, many people underestimate the extent to which their alcohol consumption contributes to their weight problem. Be very mindful of your alcohol intake throughout the week.

Portion control is especially difficult with alcohol as glasses are different sizes and hosts can be very generous. It's important to limit a glass of wine to five ounces, a beer to twelve ounces, and hard liquor to one and a half ounces per drink. (This is what constitutes a drink, as defined by the experts on alcohol consumption.) Beer really does tend to create a beer gut, so opting for wine is better.

Once you have reached your goal weight and have progressed to the Weight Maintenance part of the program, your weekly alcohol consumption can increase slightly. In chapter 8, I'll tell you how to navigate parties and other social situations where it's usually a challenge to control alcohol and food portions. Pitfalls abound when you're trying to lose weight. But don't despair, that chapter gives you strategies to avoid common traps.

Hydrate, Hydrate – with Real Water

Make sure you drink lots of water at meals and throughout the day, as well. Water helps your body function efficiently and helps you feel satisfied. While water is something we all take for granted, please stick to real water. Bottled water with added vitamins often contains a lot of sugar, and the flavored waters on the market are usually artificially sweetened. Nothing is as good for you as the real thing. (We'll get into the problem with excess sugar and artificial sweeteners later on.)

For those who don't like the taste of regular water, try dressing up a pitcher of water with slices of lemon, lime, or orange. Sparkling water can be a refreshing option as well. (Always check the label to be certain it has no added sugar and minimal sodium.)

••

Patient Story: Gaining Energy

Bernice, a thirty-eight-year-old, weighed 205 pounds (93kg), which gave her a BMI of 34 (category I obesity). Her waist circumference was 40 inches (102cm). Her LDL (bad cholesterol) was 3.46 (134 American units), and her HDL (good cholesterol) was very low at 0.84 (32 American units).

She did a lot of physical activity in her job, but did no cardio exercise. She was told that she had a significant risk of developing diabetes and heart disease due to her weight and large waist circumference. Bernice's low HDL (good cholesterol) was also a risk factor for a heart attack. The risk of becoming diabetic really scared her. Some of her friends' parents had diabetes, and she had seen them develop kidney failure due to diabetes. (One of them had to have a leg amputated.) A co-worker had died from a heart attack at age forty.

We reviewed her diet and discovered that she was eating large servings of cheese every day on her lunch sandwiches (foot-long sandwiches, packed with cold cuts). She assumed she could eat whatever she wanted because she was so young and had a physically active job.

Bernice began following the Health First program, as well as doing three other very important things.

First, she reduced her cheese consumption to only three times per week and eliminated processed meats from her diet.

Second, she separated in her mind any relationship between being physically active and food consumption. "I stopped thinking that as long as I was active, I could eat whatever I wanted. I used to think that I would just burn it off with my physically demanding job." She recognized that the way to lose weight was by eating the right foods in proper proportions.

Third, she began cardio exercise four times per week for thirty to forty-five minutes – for her health. Bernice lost 38 pounds over five months. Thanks to her exercise regime, her HDL, formerly very low, rose to a better level. "I cannot believe how much more energy I have," she said.

Eight years later, she is still 167 pounds. She power walks for forty-five minutes to an hour at least four times a week. Bernice is down to three small portions of cheese a week, has red meat just twice a week, and has stopped eating all cold cuts (processed foods). She enjoys lots of chicken, fish, and vegetables.

Bernie's risk of developing diabetes has been dramatically lowered, as well as her risk for heart disease and various cancers. Eight years later, her 38 pounds is still off. Her BMI was down to 27 (mildly overweight category), her LDL (bad cholesterol) went down to 2.4 (96 American units), and her HDL (good cholesterol) rose to 1.2 (46 American units). Her waist circumference has also decreased significantly, dramatically reducing visceral fat (fat around the organs, a dangerous fat).

Your Budget Snapshot

The Table of Threes and Fours				
3 portions per week	**4 portions per week**	**3 portions per day**	**4 portions per day**	**Unlimited servings**
Meat	Eggs	Milk, yogurt, milk alternatives*	Fruit	Vegetables
Fish		Starch (females)	Starch (males)	Poultry**
Cheese*				
* On days you have cheese, you're permitted just 2 portions of milk, yogurt, or milk alternatives.				
** For those without kidney disease.				
Note re: Alcohol				
Females: up to 4 drinks per week				
Males: up to 7 drinks per week				

4

A Recipe for Goal Attainment:

Meal Plans Made Easy

*There are only two rules for being successful.
One, figure out exactly what you want to do.
And two, do it!*

—Mario Cuomo

As forecast in the previous chapter, we turn now to seven days of meal plans incorporating the various food groups. Note that the Health First program gives you lots of flexibility in your meal choices throughout the day. You must, however, follow the budget for each food group and be vigilant with portion sizes. The last chapter ended with this Budget Snapshot. I include it here, again, as it is central to successful meal planning.

A Reminder About Portion Sizes

- One portion is generally the size of the palm of your hand for bread, pasta, rice, cereal, crackers, potatoes, couscous, and quinoa
- One portion of nuts, seeds, or fruit will also fit in the palm of your hand
- One portion of legumes is one cup

In the rest of this chapter I give a week's worth of sample meal plans.

Your Budget Snapshot – The Table of Threes and Fours				
3 portions per week	**4 portions per week**	**3 portions per day**	**4 portions per day**	**Unlimited servings**
Meat	Eggs	Milk, yogurt, milk alternatives*	Fruit	Vegetables
Fish		Starch (females)	Starch (males)	Poultry**
Cheese*				
*On days you have cheese, you're permitted just 2 portions of milk, yogurt, or milk alternatives.				
**For those without kidney disease.				
Note re: Alcohol				
Females: up to 4 drinks per week				
Males: up to 7 drinks per week				

The sample meal plans that follow are suggestions and are here primarily to illustrate how to use the budget concept. You're encouraged to build your own varied, healthy, and satisfying meals and snacks so you enjoy what you eat, avoid hunger, and lose weight.

Keep in mind, as you develop your own menus, that it is imperative to have a protein with each meal and to have an abundance of high-fiber options throughout the day. Fiber is found in whole-wheat and whole-grain starches (but you must stay within your daily starch budget), vegetables, fruits, and beans. As well as being good for you, protein and dietary fiber will satiate you longer.

SAMPLE MEAL PLANS

DAY ONE	
Meal/Snack	**Budget**
Breakfast	
Oatmeal (plain) ½ cup, made with ½ cup milk* Blueberries, handful Yogurt*, ¾ cup (cinnamon added) Coffee/tea, 1% milk but no sugar	1 starch, ½ milk/alt. 1 fruit 1 milk/alternatives
Mid-morning Snack	
Almonds, unsalted, handful	1 nuts/seeds
Lunch	
Grilled vegetables with grilled chicken	Unlimited
Mid-afternoon Snack	
Vegetables, assorted raw (Baby carrots, cherry tomatoes, yellow, red, orange peppers) Water, sparkling (low sodium)	Unlimited
Half Hour Before Dinner	
Apple	1 fruit
Dinner	
Salmon, 6oz grilled Brown rice, palm size (1 for females, 2 for males) Vegetables, stir fried (red peppers, Portobello mushrooms, onions, and asparagus) Water, lime wedge	1 fish 1 or 2 starch Unlimited
Evening Snack	
Yogurt*, ¾ cup, mixed with raspberries, handful Orange	1 Milk/alternatives 2 fruit
*0% or 1% fat variety. Remember to purchase plain yogurt with no artificial sweeteners.	

Day One Daily Total

- 1 fish
- 4 fruit
- 2 or 3 starch (depending on whether male or female)
- 2 ½ milk/alternatives
- 1 nuts/seeds

A Note About Day One

If you followed the menu as suggested, you ate well and stayed within budget in all food groups except for being short a ½ portion of milk/milk alternatives and 1 portion short on starch, which is okay.

Your Remaining Weekly Budget

- 2 fish
- 3 meat
- 3 cheese
- 4 eggs

DAY TWO	
Meal/Snack	**Budget**
Breakfast	
Eggs – 2, hard boiled, pepper (no salt) Tomatoes, red and yellow peppers Cheddar cheese, 1.5oz Coffee/tea, 1% milk but no sugar	2 eggs Unlimited 1 cheese
Mid-morning Snack	
Yogurt*, ¾ cup Almonds, unsalted, handful	1 milk/alternatives 1 nuts/seeds
Lunch	
Salad greens and assorted vegetables Grilled salmon, 6oz Oil and vinegar dressing (used sparingly) Water with lime	Unlimited 1 fish
Mid-afternoon Snack	
Strawberries, handful Cherry tomatoes, celery	1 fruit Unlimited
Half Hour Before Dinner	
Orange	1 fruit
Dinner	
Grilled vegetable salad Pasta, 3 or 4 portions with chicken and tomato-based sauce Berries, 2 handfuls Water, large glass with lime	Unlimited 3 or 4 starch 2 fruit
Evening Snack	
Yogurt*, ¾ cup, with Pistachio nuts, handful (in yogurt)	1 milk/alternatives 1 nuts/seeds
* 0% or 1% fat variety. Purchase plain yogurt with no artificial sweeteners.	

Day Two Daily Total

- 2 eggs
- 1 cheese
- 3 or 4 starch
- 1 fish
- 4 fruit
- 2 milk/alternatives
- 2 nuts/seeds

A Note About Day Two

Today you saved all your starch portions for a pasta meal, perhaps at a restaurant. You came in a little short in milk and milk alternatives, but this is allowed occasionally. Also, you went over your nuts/seeds allotment for the day, which is also allowed occasionally.

Your Remaining Weekly Budget

- 1 fish
- 3 meat
- 2 cheese
- 2 eggs

DAY THREE	
Meal/Snack	**Budget**
Breakfast	
Bread – 2 portions, whole grain with butter (sparingly) Milk*, 1 cup Coffee/tea, 1% milk but no sugar	2 starch 1 milk/alternatives
Mid-morning Snack	
Baby carrots, radishes	Unlimited
Lunch	
Roast beef sandwich 6oz lean beef, whole wheat bread, mustard, lettuce, tomato, pickle, Females: Eat this open faced Mixed green salad with assorted vegetables and vinaigrette dressing Water	1 meat 1 or 2 starch Unlimited
Mid-afternoon Snack	
Pecans, unsalted Assorted sliced raw peppers and broccoli	1 nuts/seeds Unlimited
Half Hour Before Dinner	
Banana, whole	2 fruit
Dinner	
Bowl of butternut squash soup (low salt, homemade) Grilled tilapia, 6oz Vegetables, stir-fried (snow peas, peppers, broccoli, mushrooms, and onions)	Unlimited 1 fish Unlimited
Evening Snack	
2 apples cut into small pieces Yogurt*, ¾ cup	2 fruit 1 milk/alternatives
* 0% or 1% fat variety. Purchase plain yogurt with no artificial sweeteners.	

Day Three Daily Total

- 1 meat
- 1 fish
- 2 milk/alternatives
- 3 or 4 starch
- 4 fruit
- 1 nuts/seeds

A Note About Day Three

This day had both meat and fish. You have finished your fish servings for the week.

Your Remaining Weekly Budget

- 0 fish
- 2 meat
- 2 cheese
- 2 eggs

DAY FOUR	
Meal/Snack	**Budget**
Breakfast	
Whole wheat bagel, small amount of peanut butter	2 starch
Yogurt*, ¾ cup with raspberries, handful	1 milk/alternatives 1 fruit
Coffee/tea, 1% milk but no sugar	
Mid-morning Snack	
Walnuts, handful	1 nuts/seeds
Cucumber, carrots, assorted vegetables	Unlimited
Lunch	
Turkey breast, grilled	Unlimited
Stir-fried vegetables	Unlimited
Mixed green salad with small amount of vinaigrette	Unlimited
Mid-afternoon Snack	
Mixed fruit with yogurt*, ¾ cup	1 fruit 1 milk/alternatives
Half Hour Before Dinner	
Apple	1 fruit
Dinner	
Vegetables, stir-fried	Unlimited
Chicken breast	Unlimited
Brown rice, 1 or 2 portions	1 or 2 starch
Broccoli, steamed	Unlimited
Salad, mixed greens, small amount of vinaigrette	Unlimited
Evening Snack	
Blueberries	1 fruit
Cheese, Gouda 1.5oz	1 cheese
Wine, 5oz	1 alcohol
* 0% or 1% fat variety. Purchase plain yogurt with no artificial sweeteners.	

Day Four Daily Total

- 1 cheese
- 3 or 4 starch
- 4 fruit
- 2 milk/alternatives
- 1 alcohol
- 1 nuts/seeds

Your Remaining Weekly Budget

- 0 fish
- 2 meat
- 1 cheese
- 2 eggs
- 3 alcohol (females); 6 alcohol (males)

DAY FIVE	
Meal/Snack	**Budget**
Breakfast	
All bran cereal, ½ cup Milk*, 1 cup 1 egg, soft or hard boiled Tomato slices Coffee/tea, 1% milk but no sugar	1 starch 1 milk/alternatives 1 egg Unlimited
Mid-morning Snack	
Mixture of sesame seeds, dried cranberries, dried apricots, almond slivers, handful Water	1 fruit 0.5 nuts/seeds
Lunch	
Vegetable burger, whole wheat bun with avocado spread, tomato slices, peppers, olives Milk*, 1 cup	2 starch Unlimited 1 milk/alternatives
Mid-afternoon Snack	
Yogurt*, ¾ cup (add cinnamon for flavor) Water, sparkling	1 milk/alternatives
Half Hour Before Dinner	
Pear	1 fruit
Dinner	
Steak, 6oz, lean Asparagus, grilled Spinach salad with sunflower seeds, dried cranberries, honey mustard dressing Wine, 5oz	1 meat Unlimited 1 fruit 0.5 nuts/seeds 1 alcohol
Evening Snack	
Raw vegetables with hummus dip: red, orange, yellow, and green peppers, zucchini, baby carrots	Unlimited
* 0% or 1% fat variety. Purchase plain yogurt with no artificial sweeteners.	

Day Five Daily Total

- 1 egg
- 1 meat
- 3 milk/alternatives
- 3 fruit
- 3 starch
- 1 nuts/seeds
- 1 alcohol

Your Remaining Weekly Budget

- 0 fish
- 1 meat
- 1 cheese
- 1 egg
- 2 alcohol (females); 5 alcohol (males)

DAY SIX	
Meal/Snack	**Budget**
Breakfast	
Egg, 1 hard or soft boiled	1 egg
Yogurt*, ¾ cup (cinnamon added)	1 milk/alternatives
Coffee/tea, 1% milk but no sugar	
Mid-morning Snack	
Bowl of citrus fruit, 2 handfuls	2 fruit
Lunch	
Large salad with chickpeas, kidney beans, cucumbers, carrots,	1 cup legumes
tomatoes, assorted peppers, oil and vinegar dressing	Unlimited
Water with lime	
Mid-afternoon Snack	
Pecans, handful	1 nuts/seeds
Vegetables, assorted, raw, with hummus	Unlimited
Yogurt*, ¾ cup	1 milk/alternatives
Half Hour Before Dinner	
Clementines – 2	1 fruit
Dinner	
Penne with olive oil, garlic,	3 or 4 starch
Grilled chicken	Unlimited
Vegetables, stir-fried	Unlimited
Green salad, large, calorie-reduced vinaigrette	Unlimited
Water	
Evening Snack	
Cheese, 1.5oz	1 cheese
Celery sticks	Unlimited
Wine, 5oz	1 alcohol
* 0% or 1% fat variety. Purchase plain yogurt with no artificial sweeteners.	

Day Six Daily Total

- 1 egg
- 1 cheese
- 3 or 4 starch
- 3 fruit
- 2 milk/alternatives
- 1 legumes
- 1 nuts/seeds
- 1 alcohol

Your Remaining Weekly Budget

- 0 fish
- 1 meat
- 0 cheese
- 0 egg
- 1 alcohol (females); 4 alcohol (males)

Day Seven	
Meal/Snack	**Budget**
Breakfast	
Oatmeal, plain, ½ or 1 cup, made with ½ cup milk	1 or 2 starch,
Raspberries, handful	½ milk/alt.
Milk*, 1 cup	1 fruit
Coffee/tea, 1% milk but no sugar	1 milk/alternatives
Mid-morning Snack	
Yogurt*, ¾ cup (with cinnamon)	1 milk/alternatives
Lunch	
Turkey slices (not processed)	Unlimited
Vegetables, stir-fried	Unlimited
Water with lemon	
Mid-afternoon Snack	
Vegetables, assorted raw	Unlimited
(Baby carrots, cherry tomatoes, radishes, raw turnip slices)	
Half Hour Before Dinner	
Pear	1 fruit
Dinner	
Veal medallion, 6oz	1 meat
Whole wheat couscous, 1 or 2 portions	1 or 2 starch
Asparagus, grilled or steamed	Unlimited
Bowl of berries, 2 handfuls	2 fruit
Evening Snack	
Almonds and pistachios, handful	1 nuts/seeds
Wine, 5oz	1 alcohol
* 0% or 1% fat variety. Purchase plain yogurt with no artificial sweeteners.	

Day Seven Daily Total

- 1 meat
- 3 or 4 starch
- 4 fruit
- 2 ½ milk/alternatives
- 1 nuts/seeds
- 1 alcohol

Your Remaining Weekly Budget

- 0 fish
- 0 meat
- 0 cheese
- 0 eggs
- 0 alcohol (females); 3 alcohol (males)

Note: Over the course of the week, four 5-ounce glasses of wine were consumed. This is just within the weekly limit for women, and 3 portions under for men. (During the Active Weight Loss program, women can have 4 drinks per week, and men 7 drinks per week.)

....

Patient Story: Enjoying Compliments

Sal is a thirty-six-year-old schoolteacher. He came to see me for an assessment because he was feeling sluggish. His BMI was 33, his waist circumference was high at 44 inches (112cm), and his blood pressure was elevated at 155/100. (His physical exam and blood work were otherwise normal, except that his bad cholesterol was higher than it should have been.)

A repeat blood pressure reading a few weeks later was 150/100. We talked about treatment options for his high blood pressure – medication, or weight loss and exercise, or both. His response was, "I would prefer not to start medication, but it would be easier than losing weight and exercising." I offered to teach him the Health First program to help him change his lifestyle and lower his blood pressure. He told me he wanted to think about it. He returned the next week, extremely keen to get started on the Health First program to try to control his blood pressure without medication if he could.

I asked him why he was suddenly so keen to lose the weight and change his lifestyle. He told me that, the day after our second visit, he received a call to teach a grade 1 class for a few days as a substitute teacher. On the first day, a little five-year-old girl came up to him, pushed on his abdomen with her finger, and said to him, "You're going to have a baby." He told me that upset him so much he decided to lose weight and get healthier.

Sal really committed himself to the Health First program and lost 40 pounds (20kg) at a rate of about 2 pounds (1kg) per week. His blood pressure returned to normal at 120/80. As he says:

This program is so easy to follow; I never feel like I'm on a diet, and I'm never hungry. I'm very focused on what I eat and drink. I quickly realized that I was drinking too much alcohol and eating way too many starches. Since I've lost the 40 pounds, I no longer feel sluggish, I have tons of energy, and I also like the compliments that I'm getting about how great I look. Keeping the weight off is also easy with the maintenance program that I now follow.

5

Sugar:

∙∙

More Sinister Than You Think

To eat is a necessity,
but to eat intelligently is an art.
−François de La Rochefoucauld

Now that you understand the various food groups and have started out on the weekly food plan, it's time for you to focus on what could trip you up: consumption of sugar (covered in this chapter) and consumption of salt and fat (next chapter).

Sugar consumption in our society has dramatically increased over the years. In the early 2000s, the US Department of Agriculture estimated that, on average, individual Americans consumed 90 pounds (40.8kg) of sugar per year. That's a staggering amount! All this excess sugar is a major contributor to the obesity epidemic, which, you now know, is a leading cause of diabetes, heart disease, and various cancers.

Most of the sugar we consume comes from sweetened beverages – soft drinks, energy drinks, bottled iced tea and green tea, sweetened bottled water, water with vitamins added, and special coffee drinks such as lattes, iced cappuccinos, and the like. Later in this chapter, I set out the sugar content of a long list of popular beverages that is pretty certain to shock you. It should also worry you. Recent medical information has identified sugar as a contributor to heart disease and cancer because of the way fructose is metabolized in the body. A YouTube video, "Sugar: The Bitter Truth," by Robert Lustig, M.D., reinforces our understanding of the toxicity of added sugar in our diets. In his book *Anticancer: A New Way of Life*, David Servan-Schreiber, M.D., Ph.D., implicates sugar as a cause of cancer cell growth.

A Word About High-fructose Corn Syrup (HFCS)

Sweetened beverages are popular, in part, because they are relatively inexpensive. Here's how that happened.

The 1970s saw the start of large-scale production of high-fructose corn syrup, known more commonly as HFCS. (In the UK and Canada, HFCS is sometimes called glucose-fructose syrup, and in many other countries it is also known as high-fructose maize syrup.) This byproduct of corn is intensely sweet and extremely cheap.

By the mid-1980s, HFCS was being used in a vast array of foods such as bread, cakes, pastries, pizza, and meat. HFCS also replaced sugar in soft drinks. Being 33% cheaper than sugar, HFCS was a big win for drink manufacturers but a real loss for our health.

Not only is HFCS much sweeter than sugar, but, as results from some animal studies have suggested, it may also be addictive and a significant contributor to the obesity crisis. A Princeton University research team published a report, in the *Journal of Pharmacology, Biochemistry and Behavior*, February 2010, demonstrating that rats fed HFCS gained significantly more weight than those fed table sugar, even when their overall caloric intake was the same.

You'll find HFCS in fruit juices, soft drinks, sweetened teas, specialty coffees, sports drinks, and even flavored waters. But HFCS is not found just in beverages. This inexpensive, highly potent sugar is everywhere – in cereal, breakfast bars, luncheon meats, commercial soups, bread, yogurt with fruit added by the company, ketchup, mayonnaise, and much more.

Limit your added sugar to:	
• 6 teaspoons per day *for women*	**• 9 teaspoons per day** *for men*
	Source: American Heart Association.

How to Limit Your Sugar Consumption

- Read labels
- Avoid soft drinks
- Avoid fruit juices, even unsweetened varieties
- Avoid yogurt with added fruit
- Avoid sugary breakfast cereals
- Avoid processed and packaged foods: pastries, cookies, buns, pies, ice cream

In my experience, many people don't know how much added sugar they're consuming. There appear to be two reasons for this: advertising and disclosure.

Products that contain more whole grains, fiber, and less fat are advertised to the hilt as being healthier alternatives when, in fact, these products continue to include way too much sugar. Cereal, bottled teas, and water with added vitamins are good cases in point.

Nutrition labeling is another problem. For example, sugar is cited on labels in grams – a meaningless measurement to most consumers who think in terms of teaspoons. In addition to being unhelpful, these labels can also be downright misleading. Nutrition information is often disclosed by serving size rather than for the whole container, even though people often consume the whole product as a single portion.

What Does "Added Sugar" Mean?

By "added sugar," I mean sugar that has been added to a food product. This does not include the naturally occurring sugars in fruit and milk. Most of the added sugars are to be found in processed packaged foods and beverages.

According to a 2011 Statistics Canada report, Canadian

adults and teenagers consume, on average, 26 teaspoons of added sugars per day. In a survey conducted between 2001 and 2004, the American Heart Association concluded that Americans were consuming 22 teaspoons of sugar per day. Based on a comparison of obesity rates between the two countries, I'd estimate that, if updated, the US figure would be much higher today.

Be Mindful, Read Labels, and Pay Attention to Sugars

Interpreting food labels is not always easy, but one simple tool will suddenly make grams of sugar both meaningful and actionable. Remember the number "four." **4 grams of sugar = 1 teaspoon of sugar.**

Beverages

How Much Sugar in That Soft Drink?

Here is the nutrition facts label from a 591ml (20 fl oz US) bottle of cola. Let's calculate the number of teaspoons of sugar in this popular drink.

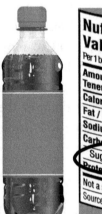
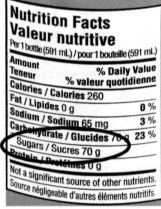

Nutrition Facts
Valeur nutritive
Per 1 bottle (591 mL) / pour 1 bouteille (591 mL)

Amount Teneur	% Daily Value % valeur quotidienne
Calories / Calories 260	
Fat / Lipides 0 g	0 %
Sodium / Sodium 65 mg	3 %
Carbohydrate / Glucides 70 g	23 %
Sugars / Sucres 70 g	
Protein / Protéines 0 g	

Not a significant source of other nutrients.
Source négligeable d'autres éléments nutritifs.

How Much Sugar in This Drink?
STEP 1: Find the sugar from nutrition facts label **70g**
STEP 2: Divide the grams of sugar by 4 to find the number of teaspoons **70g divided by 4 =17.5 teaspoons of sugar**

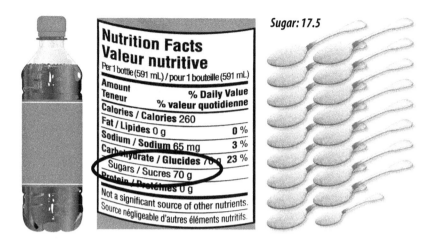

Sugar: 17.5

Nutrition Facts
Valeur nutritive
Per 1 bottle (591 mL) / pour 1 bouteille (591 mL)

Amount Teneur	% Daily Value % valeur quotidienne
Calories / Calories 260	
Fat / Lipides 0 g	0 %
Sodium / Sodium 65 mg	3 %
Carbohydrate / Glucides 70 g	23 %
Sugars / Sucres 70 g	
Protein / Protéines 0 g	

Not a significant source of other nutrients.
Source négligeable d'autres éléments nutritifs.

Imagine putting **17.5 teaspoons of sugar** on a bowl of cereal or in a large glass of homemade iced tea. The thought is enough to make you feel nauseated, but this is the amount of sugar you ingest when you quench your thirst with a 591ml (20 fl oz US) bottle of cola.

This bottle has "only 260 calories" in it. But beware – most of those calories are sugar, which is not a very healthy option. Don't be fooled by products with a low number of calories, because they may be empty and unhealthy calories.

Soft Drinks by Any Other Name: Soda and Pop

Other soft drink varieties may vary in terms of sugar content. I found a 591ml (20 fl oz US) bottle of ginger ale that contained 54 grams of sugar.

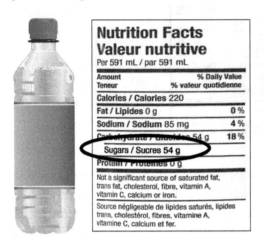

Nutrition Facts / Valeur nutritive	
Per 591 mL / par 591 mL	
Amount / Teneur	**% Daily Value / % valeur quotidienne**
Calories / Calories 220	
Fat / Lipides 0 g	0 %
Sodium / Sodium 85 mg	4 %
Carbohydrate / Glucides 54 g	18 %
Sugars / Sucres 54 g	
Protein / Protéines 0 g	

Not a significant source of saturated fat, trans fat, cholesterol, fibre, vitamin A, vitamin C, calcium or iron.

Source négligeable de lipides saturés, lipides trans, cholestérol, fibres, vitamine A, vitamine C, calcium et fer.

How Many Teaspoons of Sugar in This Drink?
STEP 1: *54g of sugar in total*
STEP 2: *54g divided by 4 = 13.5 teaspoons of sugar in the bottle*

Now imagine yourself drinking 13.5 teaspoons of sugar!

Sugar: 13.5

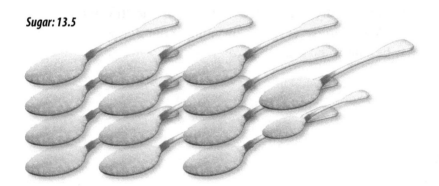

Sometimes companies try to make it appear that there is less sugar in the bottle than is really there. Here is an example.

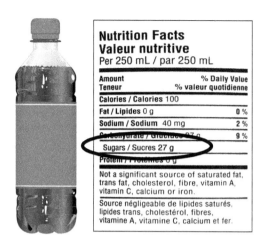

How Much Sugar?
STEP 1: Find the sugar from the nutrition facts label **27g**
STEP 2: Divide grams of sugar by 4 to find the number of teaspoons **27g divided by 4 = almost 7 teaspoons of sugar**
STEP 3: Determine the serving size (located under the nutrition facts label). As you can see, this bottle's serving size is only 250ml (8 fl oz), but the whole bottle is 591ml (20 fl oz US). You could be easily fooled to think that this whole bottle has 27g of sugar or 7 teaspoons in it, but follow along . . . **591ml (20 fl oz) divided by 250ml (8 fl oz) = about 2.4 servings**
STEP 4: Multiply the number of teaspoons by the number of servings in the bottle **7 teaspoons of sugar multiplied by 2.4 = almost 17 teaspoons of sugar in total**

Imagine putting 17 teaspoons of sugar on a bowl of cereal or in your coffee! So many people just drink and eat mindlessly. I encourage you to think before you eat and drink.

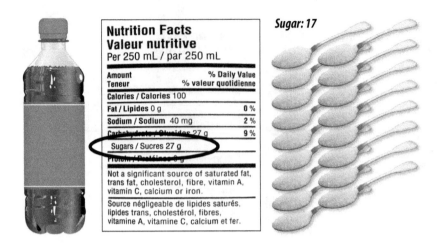

The table below provides estimates of the number of teaspoons of sugar included in many common-sized drinks found in grocery stores and restaurants.

Liquid Candy: How Much Sugar Are You Swallowing in a Soft Drink?	
Sugar quantities can vary by manufacturer and soft drink type.	
Amount*	**Teaspoons of sugar**
12 fl oz (354ml)	9.5-10.5
16 fl oz (473ml) small, fast food restaurant size	12
20 fl oz (591ml) small, movie theater size, medium fast food restaurant size	16
30 fl oz (887ml) large fast food restaurant size	24.5
40 fl oz (1182ml)	25.2
64 fl oz (1892ml) mega size at movie theaters, some convenience stores	48-54
	* Fluid ounces = US units
	Author's own consumer research.

Way Back When

In the 1950s, popular fast food restaurants offered just one soft drink size: 7 fl oz. Today, not only do they serve drinks in cups so large that you almost need a forklift to carry them, but they also permit free refills, increasing your sugar intake even more. We need to learn to stand up for our health when enticed by fast food restaurants, movie theaters, and convenience stores that wish us to purchase gigantic quantities of this liquid candy. Have water instead. No one needs a serving size nine times larger than what seemed sufficient to satisfy people in the 1950s.

Smaller Size of Container = A Great Deal Less Sugar?

Unfortunately, this is not the case. A can of popular brand cola, 355ml (12 fl oz US), looks small compared with the 710ml (24 fl oz US) and the 591ml (20 fl oz US) bottles. However, the can includes 42 grams of sugar; as you now are aware, this equates to 10.5 teaspoons of sugar (42g / 4 = 10.5).

Again, it is very deceiving if you look at only the calories in this can (160 calories), as it contains **10.5 teaspoons of sugar**.

Sugar: 10.5

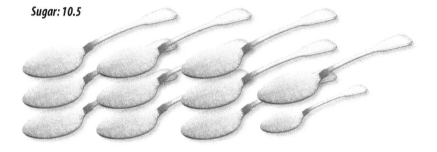

Bottled Tea

Tea has many health benefits. Green tea, in particular, includes an abundance of antioxidants. Commercially available green tea, however, can be a real sugar trap. Let's take a look at a bottle of green tea made with "natural lemon flavor."

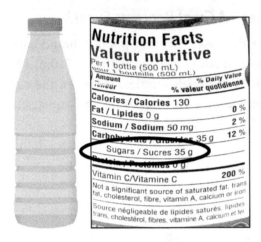

How Much Sugar in This Bottle of Green Tea?

From the nutrition facts we can see:

35 grams of sugar = almost 9 teaspoons of sugar

(The serving size is one bottle)

Sugar: 9

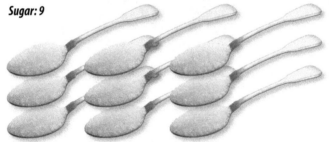

So, this "Better for You" green tea includes nearly 9 teaspoons of sugar. Don't be fooled by natural flavorings and ingredients, as there is often an overabundance of sugar.

Read Labels Carefully and Don't Be Fooled by Marketing!
Another 16 fl oz US (473ml) bottle of Lemon Tea I found says that it is made from green and black tea leaves. Sounds healthy, but the nutrition facts reveal:
36g sugar = 9 teaspoons of sugar

A 20 fl oz US (591ml) bottle of green tea with honey and ginseng boasts that it is made with 100% natural flavors, but this product includes 18 grams of sugar. Divide this by 4 and you get 4.5 teaspoons. This is high, but not astronomical until you realize that's just per cup. A 20 fl oz US (591ml) bottle contains 2.5 cups and therefore equals 11 teaspoons of sugar in one bottle.

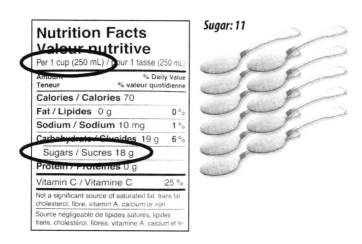

Nutrition Facts
Valeur nutritive

Per 1 cup (250 mL) / pour 1 tasse (250 mL)

Amount / Teneur	% Daily Value / % valeur quotidienne
Calories / Calories 70	
Fat / Lipides 0 g	0 %
Sodium / Sodium 10 mg	1 %
Carbohydrate / Glucides 19 g	6 %
Sugars / Sucres 18 g	
Protein / Protéines 0 g	
Vitamin C / Vitamine C	25 %

Not a significant source of saturated fat, trans fat, cholesterol, fibre, vitamin A, calcium or iron.
Source négligeable de lipides saturés, lipides trans, cholestérol, fibres, vitamine A, calcium et fer.

Sugar: 11

Bottled Water with Vitamins

As noted earlier, even water with added vitamins, the beverage industry's latest marketing innovation, has an unconscionable amount of sugar.

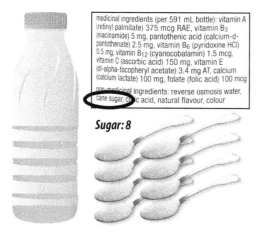

medicinal ingredients (per 591 mL bottle): vitamin A (retinyl palmitate) 375 mcg RAE, vitamin B3 (niacinamide) 5 mg, pantothenic acid (calcium-d-pantothenate) 2.5 mg, vitamin B6 (pyridoxine HCl) 0.5 mg, vitamin B12 (cyanocobalamin) 1.5 mcg, vitamin C (ascorbic acid) 150 mg, vitamin E (dl-alpha-tocopheryl acetate) 3.4 mg AT, calcium (calcium lactate) 100 mg, folate (folic acid) 100 mcg

non-medicinal ingredients: reverse osmosis water, cane sugar, citric acid, natural flavour, colour

Sugar: 8

How Much Sugar in This Water with Vitamins?
20 fl oz US (591ml) *Sugar = 33g*
33g divided by 4 = 8 teaspoons of sugar

Many people have been led to believe that this beverage is healthy, so they consume two to three bottles of this water with added vitamins per day. They are really consuming 16 to 24 teaspoons of sugar per day and, on a weekly basis, 112 to 168 teaspoons of sugar.

My advice is to stay clear of water with anything added to it. Select ordinary water and get your vitamins from a well-balanced diet with lots of fresh produce. (Sparkling water is an exception, as it has minimal sodium – salt – and no sugar.) Consider flavoring water with slices of lime, lemon, or oranges instead. Leave it overnight in the refrigerator for a refreshing drink to enjoy all day long.

Sports Drinks

Sports drinks were first developed for professional college football players. They are intended for those participating in endurance sports like running, football, soccer, prolonged cycling, long distance power walking, etc., as well as exercise in hot weather. They are high in sugar, sodium, and citric acid. This makes them effective in rehydrating your body, but they're not advisable as an everyday beverage. I suggest, if you're using one of these after an intense workout or moderate athletic activity, that you dilute the drink by 50% with water to cut down on the sugar and sodium content.

In what follows, I focus on one popular sports drink.

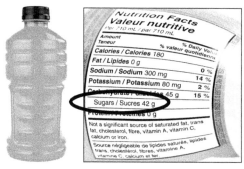

How Much Sugar in This Sports Drink?

Find the sugar from nutrition facts label **42g**

Divide the grams of sugar by 4 to find the number of teaspoons.

= 10.5 teaspoons of sugar

Sugar: 10.5

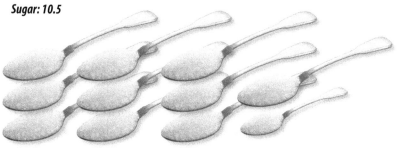

Other Popular Beverages	
Product*	**Teaspoons of sugar**
Vanilla latte supreme (med. 15 fl oz or 444ml)	4
Caramel coffee (grande, 16 fl oz or 473ml)	4
Black iced tea (grande 16 fl oz or 473ml)	5.5
Cranberry cocktail 8.5 fl oz (250ml)	5.5
White chocolate mocha 16 fl oz (473ml)	9
Iced tea (large 24 fl oz or 710ml)	15
Vanilla cappuccino (extra large 24 fl oz or 710ml)	16
Java chip specialty coffee 24 fl oz (710ml)	18.5
	* Fluid ounces = US units
	Source: Author's own consumer research.

Fruit Juice

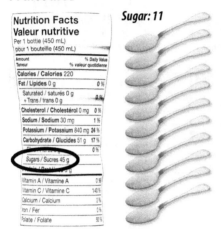

Sugar: 11

Juice most often lacks fiber, includes too much sugar, and undermines your fruit budget. Even juice made with 100% fruit and no added sweeteners should be avoided. It takes approximately eight oranges to make 16 fl oz (473ml) of orange juice. That means one cup of orange juice costs you your full daily fruit allotment and has shortchanged you of important fiber.

Don't forget, too, that the added benefit of eating your budgeted four pieces of fruit throughout the day is to help prevent hunger. You would be better to avoid juice completely.

The beverage below, made with real fruit juice, is loaded with sugar. A 250ml serving (8.5 fl oz US) has 30 grams of sugar, or 7.5 teaspoons of sugar, but actually the whole bottle is really 450ml (15 fl oz US) not 250ml (8.5 fl oz US), which is the serving size shown on the nutrition label. Therefore, there really are 13.5 teaspoons of sugar in this bottle.

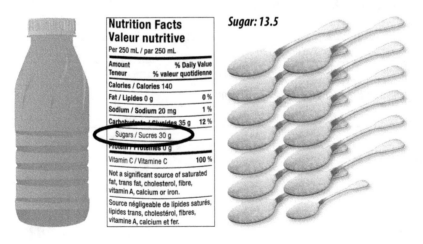

Sugar: 13.5

What About Smoothies?

With all this important news about the beverages we enjoy, can smoothies be considered healthy? The fruit and the fiber are good for you, right? Well, here again, you have to be a cautious consumer. Some commercially available products are not made with whole fruit. In fact, these should be avoided completely. Some smoothies have sizable amounts of added sugar and sodium.

Even products made with fresh fruit are problematic. The quantity of fruit they incorporate (six to twelve pieces) can send you way over your daily limit of four fruit portions. Can you imagine eating twelve fresh oranges in one sitting? I observed one product to contain two and a half mangoes, fifteen cherries, and one and a half apples in 15.2 fl oz.

If you wish to enjoy a smoothie, make it yourself with fruit that is within your budget and plain, low-fat yogurt. Unfortunately, you'll lose out on using fruit strategically through the rest of the day to manage your appetite, but, once in a while, it's a wholesome treat.

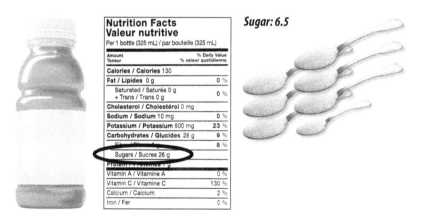

Sugar: 6.5

Nutrition Facts / Valeur nutritive	
Per 1 bottle (325 mL) / par bouteille (325 mL)	
Amount / Teneur	% Daily Value / % valeur quotidienne
Calories / Calories 130	
Fat / Lipides 0 g	0 %
Saturated / Saturés 0 g + Trans / Trans 0 g	0 %
Cholesterol / Cholestérol 0 mg	
Sodium / Sodium 10 mg	0 %
Potassium / Potassium 800 mg	23 %
Carbohydrates / Glucides 28 g	9 %
Fibre / Fibres	8 %
Sugars / Sucres 26 g	
Protein / Protéines 1 g	
Vitamin A / Vitamine A	0 %
Vitamin C / Vitamine C	130 %
Calcium / Calcium	2 %
Iron / Fer	0 %

How Much Sugar in This Smoothie?

Find the sugar from the nutrition facts label: **26g** *and divide the grams of sugar by 4* = **6.5 teaspoons of sugar** *(The serving size is one container.)*

Reduce Sugar Altogether

Now that you're aware of the gigantic quantity of sugar in many drinks, you should be working hard to cut back and ideally reduce your consumption of all sugary drinks to zero. If you're used to adding two teaspoons of sugar to your coffee, gradually reduce the amount you use so that, after two weeks, you aren't using any at all. You'll be amazed at how quickly you get used to the new taste without sugar.

Cereal

"No fat," "oat fiber," "multigrain flakes," "helps lower cholesterol." Cereal boxes make all kinds of claims to get you to pick them for your health.

Unfortunately, even cereals that include plenty of fiber and nutritious whole grains usually include three to four teaspoons of sugar per cup of cereal. Be careful here, as well, since the typical serving size on cereal nutrition labels is a ¾ or ⅔ of a cup serving. A realistic portion is 1 cup. Let's look at a few examples of "good for you" cereals.

Cereal #1

A protein and fiber cereal with a name that suggests "healthy!"

Cereal #1
- All-natural ingredients
- 7 whole grains
- 9 grams protein
- 8 grams fiber

Sounds great, right? But the nutrition facts tell a more disappointing story.

One ¾-cup serving has 13 grams of sugar = **3.25 teaspoons of sugar**	
One cup would have 16.25 grams of sugar = **4 teaspoons of sugar**	

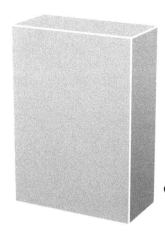

Nutrition Facts
Serving Size 3/4 cup (51 g)

Amount per serving	Cereal	With 1/2 Cup 1% Milk
Calories	210	260
	% Daily Value	
Fat 4 g†	6 %	8 %
Saturated 0.5 g + Trans 0 g	2 %	8 %
Cholesterol 0 mg	0 %	2 %
Sodium 130 mg	5 %	8 %
Potassium 160 mg	5 %	10 %
Carbohydrate 35 g	12 %	14 %
Fibre 8 g	32 %	32 %
Sugars 13 g		
Starch 14 g		
Protein 9 g		

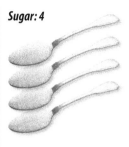

Sugar: 4

Would you put four teaspoons of sugar on your cereal in the morning?

Cereal #2

Made with whole grain and oat fiber that "helps lower cholesterol." Again this sounds like a food that will enhance nutritional health, but take a look at the sugar in the nutrition facts:

One cup has 15 grams of sugar = **4 teaspoons of sugar**

This is not as healthy as the company wants you to believe.

Cereal #3

Full of grains, raisins, and dates, with high-fiber multigrain flakes. This seems to have it all – until you turn to the nutrition facts.

One 2/3-cup serving has 10 grams of sugar = **2.5 teaspoons of sugar**
One cup would have 15 grams of sugar = almost **4 teaspoons of sugar**

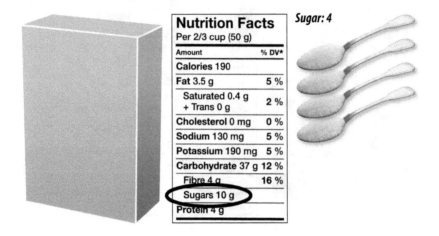

Nutrition Facts	
Per 2/3 cup (50 g)	
Amount	**% DV***
Calories 190	
Fat 3.5 g	5 %
Saturated 0.4 g + Trans 0 g	2 %
Cholesterol 0 mg	0 %
Sodium 130 mg	5 %
Potassium 190 mg	5 %
Carbohydrate 37 g	12 %
Fibre 4 g	16 %
Sugars 10 g	
Protein 4 g	

Sugar: 4

Don't be fooled by these so-called healthy cereals. Read the nutrition labels. With some searching, you can find an oat-fiber, bran, or whole grain cereal with no added sugar or with only one or two grams of sugar per cup. Add your own fresh fruit, and you have a more honestly healthy cereal breakfast.

Oatmeal

Made the old-fashioned way, oatmeal is an ideal breakfast cereal. **Oatmeal in instant packs with fruit added, however, contains three teaspoons of sugar per pack.** This is not a good choice. Instead, I suggest using the plain instant packs that have no sugar and adding your own fruit (or a very small amount of brown sugar) for a sustaining start to a great day. Or make oatmeal the old-fashioned way.

Granola Bars

Like cereal, granola bars often boast of their high fiber and whole grains, but they, too, can include far more sugar than you might suspect. Depending on the variety, the sugar content in a granola bar can be greater than that in a serving of cookies.

Granola and cereal-based bars often claim to be composed of 100% all-natural ingredients such as rolled oats, roasted nuts, dried fruit, and yogurt. They are advertised as wholesome treats, but don't be conned.

Granola Bars Versus Chocolate Chip Cookies	
Dark chocolate granola bar	13g sugar
3 chocolate chip cookies	10g sugar
Chewy granola trail mix	13g sugar
Yogurt granola bar	14g sugar

Granola bars generally are sweet snacks that serve only to cultivate your desire for more sweets. As with all products, you must read the nutrition labels carefully and be skeptical of products claiming to be good for you. Often you'll find that products have one virtue, like being low fat or high fiber, but then fall down altogether in keeping the sugar low. **Remember, 13 grams of sugar = 3 teaspoons of sugar.**

If you can't forgo the convenience of a snack bar, look for a low-sugar variety with at most four grams of sugar per whole granola bar. Keep in mind, though, that you're always better off making your own trail mix with nuts, seeds, and dried fruit. And don't overlook your other options for snacks, such as fresh fruit, low or zero-fat plain yogurt, or hummus and fresh vegetables.

Desserts

Once you wean yourself off the excess sugar incorporated into many of the foods around you, your craving for sweet foods will likely diminish. Or, at the very least, many of the foods you once craved will taste unpleasantly sweet to you. This is a good thing. Of course, you're going to want a dessert every once in a while. We're all human. The key is to make healthier choices, enjoy smaller portions, and indulge only occasionally.

It's best, while you're on the Active Weight Loss program, to completely avoid desserts, because they contain too much sugar and too many saturated fats. Each mouthful puts you a step farther from your weight-loss goal. When you move to the Weight Maintenance program (see chapter 9), you can have a dessert once a week, but in a smaller quantity than you probably had before.

You'll not feel deprived if you visualize the sheer quantity of sugar and fat in cookies, pastries, pies, and ice cream. These foods, which you may have craved in the past, undermine your health and increase your weight.

Dessert	Teaspoons of sugar
Crème caramel dessert	4
Baklava	4
Chocolate cookie	4
Honey cruller	6
Double chocolate brownie	8
Piece of lemon pie	11
Funnel cake with ice cream	11.5
Cinnamon roll	15
Piece of double chocolate cake	16.5
Bag of mints (movie theater size)	31

Source: Author's own consumer research.

Watch Out for Foods Advertised as Low Fat

I recently saw a box of ice cream drumsticks at a grocery store that proclaimed: "Vanilla and Chocolate Cone, 95% fat-free, low fat."

A look at the nutrition label shows 19 grams of sugar. Divided by four, that equals nearly five teaspoons of sugar per drumstick. Food makers often add sugar to compensate for lost flavor, courtesy of low fat. The moral here is that "low fat" doesn't necessarily mean "good for you."

Don't Be Fooled by Misleading Marketing

As with "low fat," other beneficial ingredients such as "high fiber," "whole grains," "natural ingredients," "dark chocolate," and "antioxidants," just to mention a few, can be accompanied by unhealthy amounts of sugar. Read the nutrition labels and make a defensive choice that's good for you.

Other Dairy Products	
Product	**Teaspoons of sugar**
Honey yogurt	6
Vanilla frozen yogurt	9.5
Vanilla shake (large)	22
Extra thick milkshake (large)	26

Source: Author's own consumer research.

Yogurt

Be mindful of the sugar content in yogurt. I encourage you to read the nutrition label with each yogurt purchase, either the small snack size or larger container. Most have the "fruit" added by the manufacturer, but most of that added "fruit" is mainly just added sugar in the form of syrup. For example, I recently saw a small, snack size blueberry yogurt that had 0% fat, but when I read the nutrition facts I discovered it contained 18 grams of sugar per container. As you now know, that is 4.5 teaspoons of sugar.

Nutrition Facts: Yogurt	
Sugar 18g = **4.5 teaspoons of sugar**	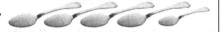

Therefore, as mentioned earlier in the book, choose low fat yogurt, plain, and add your own fruit.

Remain Mindful of Portion Size

Portion creep in commercial products has not been limited to foods such as hamburgers and fries. Desserts have also grown to be gigantic. Even when you're on the Weight Maintenance part of the program, restaurant desserts should be shared. No one can force you to eat gigantic portions.

Artificial Sweeteners

So, if sugar is to be limited for health reasons (even apart from weight loss), are artificial sweeteners okay? I wish I could say yes, but the simple answer is no! Those who drink diet beverages often do so in large quantities. Over years, that equates to a large consumption of a very unhealthy artificial product.

Although the US Food and Drug Administration and Health Canada have approved a number of sweeteners, recent studies suggest that these chemicals may increase one's desire for sweets and therefore lead to higher sugar consumption overall. Because these artificial sweeteners are many times sweeter than naturally occurring sugars (160 to 13,000 times sweeter than sugar), they are thought to trick the brain into wanting even more sweets.

Even though the science is not conclusive, it's best to stay away from artificial sweeteners altogether. My observation, in helping people lose weight, is that artificial sweeteners can be a significant barrier to their success. I encourage eating as naturally as possible – real food. If you're committed to losing weight, I recommend that you stop consumption of all diet drinks and artificial sweeteners whether in coffee, cereal, or baked goods.

I also worry that "sugar free" gives license to overindulge. Five sugar-free cookies will still give you too much fat and salt. It's not uncommon to see people ordering a diet drink with their burger and fries. They seem to feel that, because they're avoiding sugar in their drink, they can load up on salt and fat from the burger and fries.

I recommend that, instead of adding artificial sweeteners to your diet, you work on reducing the amount of sugar you eat every day. By aggressively decreasing your added sugar, you'll hardly miss it over time and ultimately will find sugary products too sweet. After about thirty days, natural flavors will seem pleasantly sweet and your desire for desserts and candies will diminish. Knowing where all the hidden sugars lurk puts you well on your way to a permanently healthier lifestyle.

The key to this chapter and better health is to:
- Read food labels for sugar content
- Remember that 4 grams of sugar = 1 teaspoon

••

Patient Story: Never Feeling Deprived

Victor is a forty-three-year-old businessman. His BMI was 35, and his blood pressure was elevated at 150/95. Victor was at risk for stroke because of his elevated blood pressure. He was at significant risk for developing diabetes, because his BMI was in the obesity category. Here is his story in his own words:

I have now lost 29 pounds using the Health First program. I feel so much better about my life. Until I started this program, I had been gaining 2 pounds every year, and I was afraid of the weight I would be at by age fifty. I no longer worry about that. I feel like I have hit the reset button.

The thing I love most about this program is that I never have to count calories. I don't ever feel deprived. Stopping all the diet pop was hard to do initially. I was drinking two Diet Cokes a day, but now I'm drinking lots of water and green tea instead. Drinking water deals with my thirst. When I want tea, I drink green tea from tea bags – no longer from bottles of green tea since I now realize these have lots of sugar. I stay away from artificial sweeteners in all drinks. I love the idea of keeping a budget for my food portions. It is so easy to do.

I use my treadmill four times a week. Exercise is now how I deal with my stress. I enjoy listening to podcasts or music with my exercise. It's "my time." I never go more than two days without using my treadmill. I just went away for a seven-day holiday with no treadmill on the property, so I just did power walking with my music every other day. Earlier in the program, I had to stay very focused, but now it's just second nature to eat this way. I'm still losing about 2 to 3 pounds per week, and will be reaching my goal weight very soon. I feel very confident that I can eat this way for the rest of my life, no question about it.

6

Fat and Salt:

The Dangerous Duo

We never repent of having eaten too little.
—*Thomas Jefferson*

We all need some fat in our diet. In fact, saturated fats help us absorb essential vitamins. However, the North American diet has too many saturated fats for good health. To improve our health, we must reduce our bad fat consumption and increase our intake of good fat.

By "bad fat," I mean saturated and trans fats. Many studies have shown that these fats contribute to heart disease, elevated cholesterol, stroke, breast cancer, colon cancer, prostate cancer, and peripheral artery disease.

By "good fats," I mean unsaturated fats (sometimes separated into mono and polyunsaturated fats). I will refer to them here simply as unsaturated fats. "Bad fats" are the saturated fats, and trans fats are the worst of the saturated fats.

Saturated Fats (BAD)	Unsaturated Fats (GOOD)
Beef	Olive oil
Veal	Canola oil
Lamb	Sunflower oil
Pork products	Peanut oil
Chicken with the skin	Sesame oil
Dairy products*	Soybean oil
Butter and lard	Corn oil
Stick of margarine	Safflower oil
Vegetable shortening	Olives
Palm and coconut oil	Almonds
Cheese	Peanuts
	Hazelnuts
	Pecans
	Cashews
	Walnuts
	Macadamia nuts
	Flax seeds
	Sunflower seeds
	Sesame seeds
	Pumpkin seeds
	Avocado

*Because dairy products are a saturated fat, I recommend dairy products with 0% to 1% fat. That way you can get all the health benefits from dairy products without consuming too many saturated fats.

Trans fats (really bad) may be in:	Fatty fishes (really good) such as:
Commercially baked:	Salmon
Cookies	Mackerel
Doughnuts	Tuna
Muffins	Herring
Cakes	Trout
Pastries	Sardines
Pizza dough	Anchovies
Packaged and Fried Foods:	Arctic char
Crackers	Whitefish (light)
Chips	
Fried foods	
French fries	
Fried chicken	
Chicken nuggets	
Breaded fish	
Candy bars	

Good Fats: But Not Too Much

All fats are high in calories, so even the good fats need to be eaten in moderation. One gram of fat has twice the calories of an equal amount of carbohydrates or protein.

Omega-3 Fats

Based on current evidence, omega-3 fats help reduce the chance of heart attack and stroke. This is a polyunsaturated fat found in cold-water fish such as salmon, herring, sardines, and mackerel. I recommend eating three servings of fish a week. Flax seed, walnuts, and canola oil are also good sources of omega-3 fats.

Healthy Oils

Oils derived from plants are better for you than lard, butter, or hydrogenated vegetable shortening, but even these oils are not equally heart-healthy. Olive oil contains the highest proportion of monounsaturated fats, with these other oils following in decreasing order:

- Olive oil (most monounsaturated fats)
- Canola oil
- Peanut oil
- Corn oil
- Sunflower oil
- Safflower oil (least monounsaturated fats)

Keep this in mind when you turn to healthy salad dressings. You may want to develop a taste for balsamic and flavored vinegars. Whenever oil is called for in a recipe, unless there is a good reason to choose otherwise, use olive oil. Oils you should avoid are those high in saturated fats, such as palm oil, coconut oil, and kernel oil.

Nuts: A Great Snack Food

Nuts are a good source of unsaturated fats, both poly and monounsaturated fats. However, you will have noted from earlier chapters that portions are not unlimited, because the calories from nuts can add up. Nuts are also a valuable source of protein. Let's look at different varieties of nuts and find out a little more about them.

Almonds	A great source of vitamin E and magnesium
Walnuts	A source of omega-3 fatty acid (the heart protection type)
Cashews	Contain lots of magnesium, oleic acid (the same healthy fat that is in olive oil)
Brazil nuts	A good source of selenium
Pistachios	Contain antioxidants and are a good source of fiber
Macadamia nuts	Slightly higher in fats and lower in protein
Peanuts	Really a legume, have the most folate
Pecans	Slightly higher in fats than other varieties

In a study in the *Journal of Circulation*, walnuts, peanuts, and pistachios all tied for first place in helping to lower LDL (bad cholesterol). Almonds were a close second. Obviously, it's important to watch your portion size when enjoying nuts. **Keep it to about a palm-sized serving per day.** Remember to pre-portion them; if you eat them directly from a container, you'll find it difficult to track the amount you have consumed. Remember, too, that unsalted dry-roasted nuts are healthier than salted ones.

Seeds: Another Healthy Snack

Seeds are a healthy snack food. The table below lists four types of seeds and their health benefits.

Flaxseed	Lots of omega-3 fatty acid (the good fat) and fiber
Sunflower seeds	Vitamin E, selenium, and magnesium
Sesame seeds	Magnesium, calcium, and zinc
Pumpkin seeds	Zinc and vitamin E

I recommend **one palm-sized serving per day.** Again, pre-portion to ensure that you don't eat a whole bag or container of seeds.

Bad Fats

Trans Fats

Why are trans fats the worst? Because they increase LDL choles-terol (the undesirable cholesterol) *and* they decrease HDL (the beneficial cholesterol). Your goal should be to reduce your trans-fat consumption to zero.

Most trans fats come from commercially prepared baked goods, margarines (especially the ones packaged as a stick), commercially prepared snack foods, French fries, and many foods prepared in restaurant and fast food outlets.

Trans fats are often listed on ingredient labels as "partially hydrogenated vegetable oil."

The vegetable oil part sounds good. It's the hydrogenation that is bad for you. Trans fats can dramatically increase the risk of developing heart disease and type 2 diabetes.

Of late, a great deal of political pressure has been brought to bear to reduce or eliminate trans fats from food, and some improvements have been made. Nevertheless, it is imperative that you read nutrition labels on all prepared foods to avoid trans fats and avoid fried foods as much as possible. I advise you to ask your server when you're in a restaurant if the kitchen uses trans fats, and then order accordingly.

Saturated Fats

Saturated fats increase the risk of heart disease, diabetes, and obesity, and they increase your LDL cholesterol. These trouble-some fats come mainly from animal meats like beef, veal, lamb, pork products, skin on poultry, and high-fat dairy products such as cheese, milk, and yogurt made with whole milk.

Avoid processed foods (which includes processed meats): they are full of saturated fats.

Fried foods, cream sauces, foods with batter, ice cream, choco-late bars, cookies, chips, and pastries, all include a great deal of saturated fats. It's best to totally avoid them during the Active

Weight Loss program. You can, very occasionally, have a small amount of one of them during the Weight Maintenance program.

Think about healthier choices, and stay within your budget. For example, given the choice between a chicken breast, a hamburger, or a piece of sirloin steak, you should choose the chicken. A 6-ounce piece of boneless, skinless chicken has about 1.2 grams of saturated fat, whereas a 6-ounce piece of sirloin steak has 5.2 grams of saturated fat. Unless it comes with nutrition facts, it's anybody's guess how much fat a hamburger contains.

Here again, nutrition labels are a valuable tool in controlling your exposure to bad fats. Read them always, and seek them out in fast food restaurants (which it would be best to avoid as much as possible). Chain restaurants have nutrition information on their websites, and now some of these restaurants even list them at the restaurant to assist consumers in identifying their healthiest menu options.

Low Fat/ Less Fat: Beware!

Be very cautious when a product states that it is low fat or less fat. Often, the product has only minimally less fat than the normal fat product. Read the nutrition facts carefully and compare it to the original product. You'll often be surprised that there is not that much less fat.

Also, don't be lulled into letting your guard down by seeing a product described as "low fat." Low fat doesn't mean you can eat large quantities of it. It's still the bad fat.

It's easy to reduce the saturated fat in your diet. Just stick to the Health First budget.

Salt (Otherwise Known as Sodium)

We all need salt to live, but the amount of sodium in our contemporary diet has become much too high. It is a significant contributor to the development of high blood pressure, which can lead to stroke and heart attack. High blood pressure is also implicated in the development of dementia and kidney disease.

On April 24, 2012, Michael F. Jacobson, Executive Director of the Center for Science in the Public Interest (CSPI), based in Washington, DC, documented in a letter to FDA Commissioner Margaret Hamburg that upwards of 100,000 lives could be saved annually if sodium levels in packaged and restaurant foods were cut in half. According to CSPI, direct medical costs in the US could be cut by about $18 billion per year if sodium consumption per person were reduced from 3400mg to 2300mg per day. This saving would increase to $28 billion if consumption were further reduced to 1500mg per day.

It's not just Americans who are loading up on salt. Health Canada estimated in 2012 that the average Canadian ingests, on average, about 3400mg of sodium per day. That is more than twice the recommended amount of 1500mg per day.

For most people, excess salt comes not so much from adding salt at the table, but from eating foods such as burgers and fries at restaurants, as well as processed sandwich meats. Processed chicken, turkey, ham, salami, and bologna are loaded with salt. Many packaged and prepared foods are also heavily salted, as are many restaurant meals.

Tips from the American Heart Association

- Eat fewer products such as salted potato chips and corn chips, lunch meats, hot dogs, salt pork, ham, dill pickles, and high-sodium canned foods
- Avoid processed, prepared, and prepackaged foods such as soups, tomato sauce, condiments, canned goods, preserved meats, and prepared mixes
- Choose lower-sodium foods, or low-sodium versions of your favorites
- Eat more fruits and vegetables. When buying canned or frozen varieties, be sure to choose the no-salt-added versions

The ideal sodium consumption limit is 1500mg a day.

To protect your health, read nutrition labels vigilantly. Look under "sodium" on the nutrition facts label. Make sure you watch for serving size when you calculate the total sodium content. For a while, anyway, try to keep track of your daily salt consumption, to make sure it's within healthy limits. Salt, like sugar, lurks everywhere. You should manage salt as diligently as you do sugar.

Sauces, gravies, and salad dressings in restaurants and stores are often very high in sodium. Even products labeled "low sodium" may be just fractionally lower than the regular versions. Be alert to this with all foods. You would be wise to avoid a food type entirely when the low-sodium version is still quite high in sodium.

At the Grocery Store
• Buy unsalted and low-sodium foods when possible
• Compare food labels. Buy products with the lowest amount of sodium
• Look for foods that have less than 360mg of sodium in a serving
• Check food labels often, because the product ingredients may change frequently, even for the same product
Eating Out
• Order smaller portions or share with someone
• Ask for gravy, sauces, and salad dressing on the side and use small amounts
• Flavor your food with lemon or pepper instead of adding salt, sauces, or gravies
• Ask for your meal to be cooked without salt or MSG, a seasoning that is very high in sodium
Source: Health Canada <www.hc/sc.gc/ca>

A 10 fl oz can of vegetable soup seems safe, comforting, and fat free, too. But look at the sodium content:

- One can contains two servings
- Sodium per serving = 770mg
- Sodium in can = 1540mg – more than an entire day's recommended limit

The Bottom Line

Fat and salt in excess undermine our health. We need a new mindset that sees value not in huge quantities of food or drink at a low price, but in fresh, wholesome ingredients that support good nutrition and don't create risks to our health.

Seek out good fats to the exclusion of others. The best way to reduce salt is to avoid fast food and processed food. Use nutrition fact labels as your best defense and, as always, keep exercising and budgeting your food groups.

• •

Patient Story: The Passion to Avoid Blindness

I am privileged to be taking care of four generations of Bata's family: Bata, her daughter, her granddaughter, and her great granddaughter. Bata is now eighty-five years old, and has had type 2 diabetes for fifteen years. She became my patient ten years ago. At that time she needed to lose about 25 pounds. Due to her weight being in the obesity category, her risk of developing the complications of diabetes, such as heart attack, stroke, kidney failure, blindness, and leg amputation, was very high. She was most afraid of going blind or having a stroke. She also wanted to avoid having to go on insulin.

Ten years ago, Bata began the Health First program with a passion. She lost 28 pounds at a rate of 1 to 2 pounds per week. She faithfully exercises three or four times a week. Her diabetes and blood pressure have been well controlled since she lost the weight and began exercising. She has not had any diabetic complications to date, despite her advanced age and her long history of diabetes, nor has she had to go on insulin. She looks much younger than her stated age and is cognitively very alert.

"I'm in better shape now than my daughter and most of my grandchildren!" she told me.

7

The Power of Moving:

Physical Activity and Exercise

*Physical fitness is not only one of the
most important keys to a healthy body,
it is the basis of dynamic and
creative intellectual activity.*

–John F. Kennedy

We all know that exercise is good for our health. Life, unfortunately, gets hectic, and time to exercise is often the first thing to go. I understand that and believe I have some tools to lead you to what I call a "Culture of Health" that will help to counter this tendency. But first, let's deal with a common misconception about exercise and weight loss.

When people want to lose weight, they generally begin an exercise program with the intention of burning fat and calories and increasing their metabolism – often without changing what, or how much, they eat. Since it is hard to lose weight through exercise alone, frustration usually sets in, and very little changes. If the same person diets, exercise will accelerate the weight reduction; however, if the person stops exercising once the desired weight loss has been achieved because they perceive the project as done, the weight will return. I would like to offer another approach that has worked with most of my patients.

Getting active and exercising should not be linked in your mind to weight loss.

View physical activity and exercise as a way, in and of itself, to improve your health. Try to separate it in your mind from weight loss. Exercise alone reduces your risk of many diseases, and improves your energy level and mental state. Yes, it will also help you lose weight, but because physical activity and exercise improve your health and well-being so much, the primary reason you do it should be for your health. Let's look at some strategies for getting and keeping your body in motion – even for those who say they don't like to exercise.

Exercise alone has been shown in many studies to decrease the risk of heart disease, stroke, breast cancer, Alzheimer's or dementia, depression, anxiety, high blood pressure, type 2 diabetes, and prostate cancer.

Physical Activity

In the Health First program, I differentiate between physical activity and exercise. Both of these are necessary for your health, physically and mentally. If you presently have little physical activity in your daily life, try to change this by walking as much as you can as part of your regular day. Following are some ideas to help you get started right now.

- Park your car at the back of the parking lot or a block away from your destination
- Walk up escalators instead of just standing on them, or better yet, use the stairs
- Get off the subway or bus one stop early
- Take stairs for a floor or two instead of the elevator
- Take a walk at lunch time and/or after dinner
- Take walks throughout your day of two to three minutes each
- Take a roundabout route to common destinations
- Never use drive-through services

- Have seasonal footwear in your car so you can go for a walk when you find yourself early for an appointment
- Walk the golf course – all eighteen holes, or just nine holes to start
- Work in your garden
- Play street hockey
- Go for bike rides
- Go roller blading

There's no doubt that being more active is going to require a little more time out of your day, but it is guaranteed to improve your health. Try getting up earlier to spend, as a start, ten to fifteen minutes walking on a treadmill. Drive to work twenty minutes earlier and walk around the building. Take a longer walk with the dog, or take a longer way to get to your mailbox if you don't have home delivery. You could start a walking group with your workmates or neighbors to make use of time available at lunch or after dinner. Meet a friend early in the morning and go walking. On weekends, you could encourage your partner, friends, and/ or children to keep you company as you power walk around the neighborhood.

Moderately paced walking helps bones retain their strength. Osteoporosis is a condition in which bones become brittle, often due to inadequate weight-bearing physical activity such as walking. **Walking is one of the best ways to help prevent osteoporosis.**

Speaking of steps, it's a good idea to count your steps. I recommend to many of my patients that they buy a pedometer. I encourage them to work up to 5,000 to 10,000 steps a day. This goal may seem ambitious, but once you start, you'll enjoy the daily challenge this creates. You can do it. You'll be surprised how much more energized you'll feel right away.

Regular walking for at least 30 minutes per day has been shown to reduce the risk for type 2 diabetes by 35-40%, according to the International Diabetes Federation.

Shape Up!

A program called Shape Up America! – founded by former US Surgeon General C. Everett Koop in 1994 – recommends 10,000 steps every day. Here's how you can do this (from <www.shapeup.org>):

- Have good walking shoes and replace them regularly
- Wear a pedometer for two weeks without changing your normal activity
- Log your steps every day
- Take the highest number you have walked in that time (if you're comfortable with that) and use it as your daily goal for the next two weeks
- After two weeks, review your log and determine if you're ready for 500 more steps
- Add comfortable increments every two weeks or longer, if necessary, until you have reached 10,000 steps daily. Check with a physician if you experience pain that concerns you

---

Pedometers and You

These inspiring little devices can be purchased for $10 to $20 at many stores and are also easily available online. Go slowly at first, if you're not used to being physically active. Even walking five to ten minutes four times a week will help you feel great. Then gradually build up to longer walks and add in exercise.

It is estimated that if you are inactive and then become physically active you can reduce your risk of heart attack by 35% to 55%.*

---

* Heart and Stroke Foundation of Ontario (3/6/2012).

Exercise

When I talk about exercise in the Health First program, I mean cardio exercise. In addition to consistently trying to increase your physical activity, you still need cardio exercise to dramatically reduce your risk of disease. **I strongly recommend that everyone gradually work up to from thirty to forty-five minutes of moderate-intensity cardio (aerobic) exercise four times per week.** Start slowly and work up to this level. The amount of time this will take depends, of course, on the level you're starting from.

Note: Before starting any exercise program, first check with your physician to ensure that you're able to do regular exercise. If you haven't been physically active, start slowly with five to ten minutes, four times per week, and build up to your goal. Always warm up before you exercise.

A short time after you start an exercise program four days per week, you'll notice you have more energy, better concentration, a greater sense of well-being, an improved mood, and better sleep. For some, this happens very quickly, while for others, it takes a little longer. Diabetics find that their blood sugars improve with exercise. Patients with high blood pressure find that their readings get better, too.

Regular cardio exercise not only will reduce your risk of getting many common cancers, but also, if you have had breast cancer, prostate, or colon cancer, for example, a cardio exercise program may help to reduce your risk of recurrence. Cardio exercise is also a tremendous way to reduce stress.

Patients often ask what kind of cardio exercise I recommend. My overall answer is, "Whatever you think you would most enjoy." Here, nevertheless, are some specific suggestions:

- Power walking outside or on a treadmill
- Running on a treadmill (or outside)
- Exercise bike
- Elliptical machine
- Rowing machine

- Stepper
- Aerobics class
- Team sports like volleyball, hockey, soccer, basketball
- Aqua-fit
- Spinning class
- Stair climbing
- Swimming

Exercising with a friend is usually more fun and helps to keep you motivated.

Team sports are worth considering, as long as you can get sufficient playing time. Mix up your exercise, too, to find what you like best and to avoid boredom.

Intensity

What should your goal be in terms of exercise intensity? There are a number of methods for measuring exercise intensity. Here are two approaches I suggest.

The Huff and Puff Rule
Gradually build up to thirty to forty-five minutes of huffing and puffing such that it is challenging to talk at the same time. (But not to the point where you're unable to talk.)
Heart Rate Target
To determine your ideal heart rate target (pending your own physician's approval), use the following standard unisex formula: (220 − your age) x 60% **As your fitness level improves, you can gradually increase your heart rate target to a maximum of 85%.**

You can determine your heart rate by using a heart rate monitor, or by counting your pulse for ten seconds and multiplying that by six to get your rate for a full minute. You can find your pulse on the outer edge of your wrist or use the carotid pulse in your neck.

EXAMPLE: Mark is a healthy fifty-year-old man. His initial target heart rate would be: 220 – 50 = 170   170 x .6 = 102 heartbeats per minute
Mark should work up to a target heart rate of: 220 – 50 = 170 and 170 x .85 = 144 heartbeats per minute

Whether you use the simple Huff and Puff Rule or the Target Heart Rate method, work up to your exercise goal at a comfortable, sustainable pace.

The Canadian Diabetes Association reports that regular physical activity improves your body's sensitivity to your natural insulin and helps manage your blood glucose levels.

If you're not used to exercising, begin slowly. Begin by increasing your physical activity, and then move into short sessions of cardio exercise, starting at five to ten minutes, four days a week. Gradually increase to thirty to forty-five minutes, four days per week. The first few days of exercise will be the hardest. After that, you'll find your improvements to be exponential and the benefits to be astonishing.

In my opinion, it doesn't matter what time of the day you choose to exercise. Mornings work for some, while afternoons or evenings are better for others. Do what works best for you. Remember – there are seven days in a week; exercising just three or four days out of the seven will dramatically change your life. You're likely to identify many barriers or excuses for skipping exercise. Let me offer several tools to help you power on.

Your Exercise Toolkit

Exercise Buddy

I encourage you to find someone to exercise with. Power walk with a friend, join a power walking group or a running group, play squash, or go regularly to an aerobics class or spinning class at your local community center, YMCA, or gym. The socialization and sense of community that often develops will make the exercise seem less tedious. And the other benefits – new friendships and increased energy and well-being – will motivate you to keep exercising.

Linkage

Link exercise with something you enjoy and are already doing. If you like watching TV, do so while you use a treadmill, stationary bike, elliptical machine, or rowing machine for forty-five minutes. If movies are your passion, watch the first hour while you're on your treadmill. A patient of mine liked to watch a lot of sports events on TV. He decided he would watch these events only if he was on the treadmill. Most libraries allow free downloads of audio books in MP3 format, which is great entertainment while power walking. Assembling a collection of your favorite upbeat music can make exercise an enjoyable time to listen to music.

Scheduling

There is ample scientific evidence that regular exercise dramatically reduces the risk of developing a large number of diseases. So why aren't we all exercising? The most common reason I hear for failure to exercise is "not enough time." I respect and understand this – we all live busy lives. Yet we schedule things every day – meetings, dinner with friends, a baseball game, dentist or doctor appointments, hockey practices, ballet or karate classes for the kids, and so on. We all schedule things we want to accomplish because scheduling works. That's why I offer you these two simple rules that will definitely help you incorporate exercise into your life and make it a permanent part: "Just book it" and "Just do it."

"Just Book It"

I recommend that, every Sunday night, you book three or four exercise appointments for the next seven days of your life. Book your appointments for whenever they fit your schedule for that week. If Thursday, Friday, Saturday, and Sunday work for you, that's okay. The most important thing is to get three or four sessions completed per week. Even if the times and days for exercise vary from week to week, promise yourself three or four workouts a week.

Use the same scheduling devices for your exercise that you

currently use to schedule your other appointments – your iPhone, Blackberry, Android, Gmail calendar alert, appointment book, calendar – whatever it takes to keep you on track.

One of my patients traveled to Russia on business for five days. He had already booked his workout time in the exercise room from 7:00 to 7:45 a.m., Monday to Thursday inclusive. To his dismay, the exercise room at his hotel was closed for renovations. So strong was his resolve to be true to his exercise program, however, that he immediately rebooked his appointments to a time that week when he would be home. He exercised faithfully on Saturday and Sunday from 8:00 to 8:45 a.m. and from 4:30 to 5:15 p.m. both days, times when his family was least likely to notice his absence.

This was not his ideal approach to exercise, but for that particular week he just did it, achieving his goal of always exercising four days a week for his health.

"Just Do It"

All the greatest plans and ambition to exercise fall short without this one simple rule: **Just do it ... never cancel.**

When something is important to us, we keep our commitment to it even when we don't feel like following through. You wouldn't think of skipping a scheduled meeting with your boss or a colleague, even if you were knee-deep in work. The kids have to be picked up from lessons even when you feel like staying on the couch. You keep a doctor's appointment, or a promise to meet a friend to help with a problem, even when time to yourself might be more appealing.

I highly recommend that you give exercise the same priority and obligation level as the other important responsibilities in your life – even if you feel tired. Never cancel your exercise appointments.

Use Your Toolkit

There's a popular perception that staying committed to an exercise program requires great discipline. I don't believe it does. All it requires is following two simple rules: **Just book it** and **Just do it**. Would you say it takes discipline to stop at a red light and go when it turns green? We all respect traffic signals, which shows that following rules is quite different from summoning up discipline. I suggest that you try exercising regularly for thirty days and see just how well it works.

There's no doubt that it's hard to place exercise as a top priority in an already crowded life, but think of it this way: without your health, everything could change. You might not be able to work or go to school or enjoy family and friends.

I believe it is truly worth the effort to exercise regularly and consistently, and to incorporate physical activity into daily life.

Once you truly believe that regular exercise is critical for your health, and commit to reducing your risk of developing diabetes, heart disease, Alzheimer's, breast cancer, and many other diseases, these tools will change your life forever. You'll move forward toward what I call a culture of health and enjoy a sense of empowerment. You'll be taking charge of your health and your future.

Exercise: Book It and Just Do It

- *Every Sunday night, schedule three or four exercise appointments with yourself for the following week. Use any scheduling tool you normally use for all your appointments (Scheduling)*
- *Treat these appointments as mandatory, whether you feel like it or not when the time arrives (Priority scheduling)*
- *Get your family and friends involved for encouragement and mutual benefit (Exercise Buddy)*
- *Make exercise time fun. You want to look forward to exercise in order to diminish excuses (Linkage)*
- *Ideally, exercise four times per week, working up to forty-five minutes per session*
- *Default: four times a week for thirty minutes, three times a week for forty-five minutes, or three times a week for thirty minutes*
- *Double Up: You can do one hour of exercise on one day to equal two sessions out of the ideal of four sessions per week. You could also break it up into two half-hour*

*sessions the same day; for example, do cardio on Saturday morning for thirty
minutes and then again on Saturday afternoon for thirty minutes for two sessions
in one day. If life gets busy and you find you can exercise only on the weekend, make
sure you get in a minimum of three thirty-minute sessions. While this is not ideal,
at least you'll have completed the minimum. In the example above, you would
just need to do one thirty-minute exercise session on Sunday to accomplish your
minimum of three thirty-minute sessions per week*

- *Always strive daily to do as much walking as you can to attain the goal of
5,000 to 10,000 steps per day*

Warning: Don't Fool Yourself with Calorie Burn

Many exercise machines, and even some computer programs,
give you a tally of the total calories you're burning during exercise. Perhaps the designers think this is encouraging. I believe it is
misguiding. I don't trust the calculators to be accurate.

Furthermore, I feel that this practice can be counterproductive.
For example, if your treadmill flashes a burn of 500 calories, it's
easy to say to yourself, "Now I can have a piece of cake." You figure
a piece of cake is about 250 calories and that you're still ahead
by 250 calories. Not true. The original calorie burn was almost
certainly exaggerated, and the calorie content of your dessert is
likely underestimated.

Trusting these readings becomes even more misguided if you
eat more at a meal than you should and justify it by promising
yourself that you'll burn it off the next day. It is very hard to exercise away overindulgence. Exercise doesn't burn as many calories
as you think.

In my opinion, playing the calorie game is no way to live. It's a
game you're always going to lose. I cannot stress enough that you
should exercise for good health, to give yourself more energy, to
reduce your stress, and to reduce your risk of disease. It can be very
liberating to disconnect exercising from burning calories.

A Culture of Health

Health will become a bigger part of your mindset as you incorporate exercise and physical activity into your life, even if you don't enjoy it at first. You'll discover yourself making healthier choices with food, sleeping better, and reducing your stress through exercise. If you smoke, you may even be motivated to quit smoking to make your cardio workouts less difficult. As you adopt this culture of health, you may find that other people around you – children, partners, co-workers, and friends – start to join in. You'll find yourself seeking out others who share this passion. It's a mindset that generates community.

A Word About Resistance Training

Although I feel resistance training is important, I recommend, with the Health First program, that you initially focus on increasing your daily physical activity and then work to increase (gradually if necessary) your cardio exercise to four times per week for forty-five minutes. (Remember, it's important for you to stretch for ten to fifteen minutes after you finish your cardio exercise to prevent injury.)

Once you've embraced this program and have achieved your weight-loss goal, you can start to incorporate some resistance and weight training into your exercise program. I suggest two days a week for fifteen to thirty minutes. My experience with patients is that this order of exercise sequencing works best.

With a commitment to being more active every day and exercising four days a week, you're on your way to a personal culture of heath.

....

Patient Story: When Health Becomes Second Nature

Debbie, a seventeen-year-old, was concerned about her weight, as she was going off to university the following year. She weighed 170 pounds (77.5kg). She was doing very little exercise, and was not very mindful about what she was eating. She wanted to lose weight, but didn't want to go on any fad diets, as so many of her girlfriends had tried them, lost weight, and then gained it all back.

She embraced the Health First program, consistently lost 1 to 2 pounds per week, and reached her target weight loss of 28 pounds. She made exercise a part of her life, and focused on being physically active every day. Now, at age twenty-five, she has kept her 28 pounds off, goes to the gym three or four times a week, and follows the Weight Maintenance part of the program religiously. As she puts it:

I got it! It is now just second nature to me to stay focused, eat healthy foods in proper portion sizes, and exercise. It's that simple. I see my co-workers eating junk food at work. I bring lots of vegetables, have my four fruit portions per day, and eat three healthy meals a day, along with four snacks. I will often go to the gym at 5:00 p.m. and then come back to the office to finish my work.

8

Staying on Track:

000000000000000000000000000000000000000

Avoiding Common Pitfalls

Take the first step in faith.
You don't have to see the whole staircase,
just take the first step.
—Dr. Martin Luther King Jr.

While you're revamping your lifestyle, your determination may waver. That is natural and to be expected. It's important, at these low times, to remember that you're doing this for a greater purpose than simply losing weight. You're doing this for your health and your happiness.

Fundamentally, you must believe in yourself and your power to build new and better habits. Motivation and determination need to be matched with a few effective strategies.

I close this book, therefore, with a powerful way for you to stay on track with the Active Weight Loss part of your program. Then I help you steer clear of common pitfalls. Finally, I give you one simple trick for the Weight Maintenance part of your program – maintaining your success. It is challenging to lose weight, become more physically active, and exercise regularly, but, with the help of certain techniques, it's not as difficult as you might think.

The Steps for Success

It may be true that a journey of a thousand miles begins with a single step, but how do you make that very first step when you know how challenging the goal is? Say you have 40 pounds (18kg) to lose. That may seem overwhelming and discouraging, especially if you've tried other programs unsuccessfully in the past.

Cast out all those negative thoughts. Everything must start small, like a bird's nest from a single strand of grass. The key to losing weight (and becoming more active) is to focus on small, achievable goals – what I call the steps for success.

Set your mind on losing just 10 pounds (4.5kg). Give yourself five to eight weeks to accomplish this, but strive to lose 2 pounds (1kg) each week. Similarly, try to set a physical activity goal of 5,000 to 10,000 steps per day. And, equally important, gradually increase your cardio exercise to forty-five minutes, four times a week. You should not try to lose more than 2 pounds per week, as crash dieting does not result in sustainable weight loss.

Modest, credible goals wedded to regular habits will be your lifelong partner for good health.

The First Step of Success
10 lbs (4.5kg) @ 2 lbs (1kg) weight loss per week

Break down your weight-loss goals into achievable steps. Focus on losing just 10 pounds (4.5kg) at a rate of about 2 pounds (1kg) per week.

Once you've succeeded at your first step, you'll have lost 10 pounds (4.5kg), a significant amount of weight loss that will result in a real improvement in your health. As you reach your second step, you'll be on your way to dropping 20 pounds (9.1kg), which will create a tremendous health benefit. Continue building ten-pound steps until you've reached your goal.

The Second Step of Success
10 lbs (4.5kg) @ 2 lbs (1kg) weight loss per week

Now 20 pounds gone!

Step on Your Scale Weekly

Goals are great, but results are what really matter. **Weigh yourself every Monday morning, just after you wake up.**

Ideally, you will want to observe a weight loss of 2 pounds (1kg) each Monday morning, but if you have lost less than that, don't be discouraged. If you have lost 1 pound (0.5kg), then you're still moving in the right direction, which is better than where you were before. If you didn't lose any weight, or if you gained, try to analyze why and make the necessary corrections to achieve better results the next week.

Believe in yourself and don't give up.

Be positive. Be mindful every day. Frequently, especially at the beginning, review the components of the diet every morning. The best way to lose weight is to practice good eating habits every single day.

Helpful reminders:

- It is most important to follow the Health First program to the letter
- Don't become discouraged if you do not reach your weekly goal
- Believe in yourself
- Stay focused and mindful every day
- Remember, you're doing this for your health

Pitfalls and Tools

Like anything that is challenging, many social and psychological situations may intervene to throw you off track. Be kind to yourself, but be on guard. Learn from your slip-ups, and immediately get back on the program. Here are common pitfalls you may encounter while forging ahead to a healthier you.

"I Didn't Know!"

By now you have probably discovered that some regular foods that you thought were perfectly wholesome can undermine a healthy diet. Who knew that some granola bars could be so high in saturated fat and sugar? And that yogurt with fruit added by manufacturers contains a ton of sugar?

I cannot emphasize enough how important it is to read nutrition labels. This instant information will prevent you from falling into the biggest pitfall of all – not knowing. Always be curious about ingredients and nutrition facts. Be vigilant. The ingredients in products that you know can change, for better or worse.

Hunger

Very simply, never let yourself get hungry. Have three regular meals each day and snack strategically. Drink water. Be mindful of snack times, and take snacks with you when you're out so you don't come home ravenous. If you don't have a snack with you, stop and buy a nutritious one.

At home, always have lots of healthy snacks within easy reach, including fruit, yogurt, nuts, fresh cut-up vegetables, and hummus. It's best, during the Active Weight Loss program, to keep foods such as chips, cookies, and ice cream out of the house so you do not undermine your success.

Parties and Social Functions

I recommend always eating a piece of fruit half an hour before attending a social gathering so you don't arrive hungry, potentially causing you to reach for unhealthy foods. If you know the event will involve snacking instead of a full meal, have a well-balanced meal first and consider taking your own plate of cut-up vegetables.

When a meal is being served, find out in advance what will be on the menu. If meat is the main course and you've already had your limit of red meat for the week, just ask for a different protein, such as chicken or fish.

As for potluck meals, it's always a great idea to take vegetable appetizers or a fruit dessert to help you stay on track.

At social functions and other multi-course occasions, you can and should refuse dessert and any other serving that will undermine your daily and weekly budget. Before the meal service starts, ask for salad with the dressing on the side and ask to have cream sauces left off your plate. Wait staff can easily accommodate this kind of simple request. You might even want to phone ahead to find out what's on the menu so you can accommodate the function within your weekly food budget.

Patients tell me that they are sometimes pressured by friends or family to eat things they are trying to avoid. If you're ever in this situation, don't mention that you're on a diet – just explain that you're just trying to eat healthier.

At a fundraising gala, one of my patients asked the organizer what was being served and was told that it was roast beef. She asked for a fish dinner instead, without cream sauce. The organizer was only too happy to help.

Another patient found that her mother-in-law felt slighted when she did not eat the large portions she was served. But she understood when my patient explained that her doctor was helping her lose weight to avoid diabetes.

Buffets

The big trouble with buffets is that most of us feel we have to get our money's worth. We pile on the food because it's there, it looks great, and it gives us value for money. This is, of course, self-defeating. The real value in food is its health benefits. You get the maximum value out of a buffet by eating in a healthy way, which means loading your plate with vegetables and a normal portion of fish or grilled chicken. Whenever you're confronted with an over-abundance of food, ask yourself how you can get the most benefit out of your meal by taking only what will keep you healthy and satiated.

Portion size matters. Smaller is healthier. Bigger is not.

Emotional Eating

We all tend to eat when we're bored, depressed, anxious, or in need of comfort. Beware of this tendency. Try to be mindful – don't allow emotions to dictate what you eat. Make every effort not to use food as a way of coping with emotions. Instead, distract yourself. Call a friend, go for a walk, or get on a treadmill. Recognize your emotions and give yourself permission to have them, but don't allow them to undermine your major health goals.

If you feel you simply must eat to relieve stress, munch on some chicken leftovers, or, better yet, go for nature's best finger foods: apples, cherry tomatoes, celery, carrots, or sweet peppers cut into wedges.

Not Getting Enough Sleep

Many studies have shown that people who get adequate rest are more successful in losing weight. The world is a whole lot rosier when a good night's sleep has given you the energy to eat right and exercise well. I strongly advise getting seven to eight hours of sleep each night. This will definitely enhance your weight-loss success.

Slip-ups

You may have a slip-up and revert to old eating habits. Don't beat yourself up if this happens. Just get right back on track with the next snack or meal. It's a good idea to analyze why it happened and to take steps to prevent it from happening again. Be supportive of your efforts to get healthier and be your own best support team.

Controlling Portion Sizes

Focus on portion size, especially when going out to eat. Some tricks that can help are to:

- Share the appetizer and the entrée – sharing is caring
- Order a luncheon size, if possible, when out for dinner
- Order an appetizer size of the entrée you want, then ask for extra vegetables or a larger salad

One of my patients told me a great way to deal with portion creep. His job required him to entertain clients who frequently wanted to go to Italian restaurants. When his pasta dish arrived, he asked the waiter to immediately box half of it. Not only did this keep him from eating the whole large portion, but it also gave him a great deal – two meals for the price of one. At home, make every effort not to put serving dishes on the table, or, if you must, be sure to keep the serving dish at the other end of the table so it takes effort to get it. Eat lots of extra vegetables, and, if you're really hungry, have an extra piece of fish or chicken.

Patient Story: Determined to Prevent Diabetes

In January 2007, Geraldine, at age fifty-four, had a BMI of 32.5 and a waist circumference of 38 inches (96cm). Both these measurements placed her at significant risk of diabetes, stroke, and several cancers, including breast and uterine cancer. Her blood sugar was in the pre-diabetic range. "I'm terrified of getting diabetes," she told me.

Geraldine embraced the Health First program with tremendous enthusiasm, determined to prevent herself from getting diabetes. She lost 34 pounds, at 2 pounds per week. Her blood sugar returned to normal, and she now feels very confident that she will never succumb to these chronic diseases. She has maintained all but 3 pounds of her 34-pound weight loss. She weighs herself every day, does cardio exercise four days a week, and always stays focused on what she is eating. She told me just recently that she feels so much younger than her friends of the same age.

9

Maintenance:
∙∙∙
Sustaining Your Achievement for Life

Optimism is the faith that leads to achievement.
Nothing can be done without hope and confidence.
—Helen Keller

Patient Story: Avoiding More Pills

Harry, a seventy-one-year-old, was diagnosed with type 2 diabetes some years ago by another physician, who urged him to go on diabetes medication. Already taking pills for high blood pressure, he did not want to take more medication. I advised that he could either start medication to get his blood sugar into the target range or lose 50 pounds to get out of the obesity category and get his blood sugar into the normal range.

Determined to avoid more pills, he embraced the Health First program's diet and exercise regime and did extremely well. He became "obsessed" with power walking four days a week for forty-five minutes. He lost 50 pounds, at a rate of about 2 pounds a week. His blood sugar returned to the normal range, and he accomplished his goal of not having to take medication for his diabetes.

He said he felt a sense of victory over his diabetes. Six years later, his blood sugar is still in the normal range, and his 50 pounds are still off. He is very physically active and continues to exercise as he follows the Health First Weight Maintenance program.

Keeping the Weight Off

During the Active Weight Loss part of the Health First program, I encourage patients to aim to lose 1 to 2 pounds (about 0.5kg to 1kg) per week. It is important, once you have achieved your personal weight-loss goal, to engage in the Weight Maintenance program to sustain your weight loss.

Some simple rules will help you to avoid gaining the weight back, something that happens to many people who do not engage in a maintenance program. Of course, maintaining your weight loss will help you reduce your risk of getting a variety of diseases.

To maintain your desired weight, you need to continue your new lifestyle of eating healthy, watching portion control, and staying mindful and focused on what you're eating as well as engaging in daily physical activity and doing cardio exercise three or four times per week. To sustain your weight loss, it is critically important to view your newly adopted lifestyle as a transformation in the way you live.

I recommend making some minor adjustments in your weekly food budget to maintain your weight loss and prevent any further loss once you're at your target weight. **The maintenance program allows one extra starch portion per day (be sure that it is whole wheat, whole grain, or brown rice).** I highly recommend that you continue with your budget of only three meat portions and three cheese portions per week, as moving beyond this increases your intake of saturated fats too much, which then increases your risk of colon cancer, breast cancer, heart disease, or stroke. Of course, your weight will go back up as well.

Portion Creep

Be vigilantly mindful of portion size, as portion creep continues in restaurants and packaged foods unabated. Using the palm of your hand as your measuring device will allow you to stay on track and not gain your weight back.

Desserts: One per Week

During the Weight Maintenance program, it is okay to have one dessert per week, and I usually recommend that you treat yourself over the weekend. However, continue to pay attention to portion size. Have a small portion of dessert or share the dessert with your partner or friends. I strongly urge you, if you used to eat a lot of desserts, to avoid going back to that way of life. Try to think of dessert as a great deal of sugar and saturated fats, which you can partake in once a week as a treat. Remember, you can use one of your fruit portions for a "dessert."

> Another critical step in maintaining your awesome weight loss is to weigh yourself first thing every morning, just after you wake up.

I know that, for some people, this sounds obsessive, but you cannot change and adjust what you do not measure accurately.

I have found that daily weighing is the single most important step in my patients' success in sustaining their weight loss. Allowing a 1 to 2 pound (0.5 to 1kg) swing in your daily weight is okay, but when it moves beyond this, you should immediately swing into the Active Weight Loss program until you have achieved your target weight once again. I cannot emphasize enough the importance of this one simple step to prevent gaining back your weight.

Additionally, if you find that your weight goes up beyond the 1 to 2 pound (0.5 to 1kg) limit, try to analyze the cause and retake the steps you followed to lose the weight in the first place until you're back to your target weight. It simply works.

Slip-ups

Holidays, weddings, family celebrations, birthday parties, weekends away, conferences, business trips, and the like put us at risk of weight gain. Staying mindful and not overindulging will help to prevent swings in your weight.

Remember the tools that are available to you:

- Eat healthy snacks mid-morning, mid-afternoon, and a half-hour before dinner and in the evening
- Drink a glass or two of sparkling water between each alcoholic drink at social events to reduce the amount of alcohol you consume

However, if you find that you have gained three pounds, *immediately* get back on the Active Weight Loss program, and within a very short time, you'll be back to your goal weight again. With your goal weight achieved once again, you can move back into the Weight Maintenance program.

Life is to be enjoyed, so don't be too hard on yourself if you slip up, which very well may happen. The most critical step is to get back to the Active Weight Loss program and restore your weight back to your goal. Only with accurate daily measurement can you be 100% aware of what your weight is and take action immediately before it gets out of control.

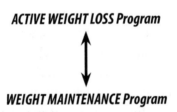

ACTIVE WEIGHT LOSS Program

WEIGHT MAINTENANCE Program

A balancing act between maintenance and active programs will help you keep your yourself at goal weight.

When most people think of losing weight and dieting, they think they will feel deprived and be required to sustain a very restricted life. As you'll find, the Health First Active Weight Loss part of the overall program does not require you to live this way to be successful at losing weight and becoming healthier. And, what's even better is that the vast majority of my patients have not gained their weight back because they have adopted a new lifestyle: eating healthy foods, being mindful of portion size, consulting their food budget, and participating in physical activity and exercise as a permanent change in their lives.

Maintaining Your Weight Loss
• Weigh yourself every morning
• Eat healthy food
• Be mindful of portion size
• Adhere to your food budget
• Be physically active and exercise

When they do gain a few pounds, they see the increase on their scale and get back on track quickly. In my experience, when people gain more than 3 pounds (2.3kg), those 3 pounds can quickly become 7 pounds, then 10 pounds, and, before they know it, they have gained most of their weight back.

By doing the **ACTIVE WEIGHT LOSS ⟷ WEIGHT MAINTENANCE dance**, you'll find it much easier to stay on track. And, like most of my patients, you'll keep your weight off for life.

Life Gets in the Way

So far, I've focused mainly on slip-ups in the diet. Another key factor in maintaining your weight-loss success is a daily focus on being as physically active as you can, always striving for that 5,000 to 10,000 steps per day *and* always "booking those cardio exercise appointments" and "doing it."

Patients tell me that, in addition to daily weighing, the best way to maintain weight loss is to engage in physical activity and cardio exercise. Most people find that, over time, they feel sluggish and tired if they do not exercise three or four times a week. I personally share these feelings and just don't have as much energy if I'm not exercising three or four times per week.

You Are in Good Company

The vast majority of people who have participated in this program keep the weight off. You also can accomplish this second major success – maintaining your weight loss. You now have the skills to prevent yourself from slipping back. Don't sell yourself short. You can be successful in maintaining your new-found freedom. If you start to slip, remember to just pick up this book again and review as much of the material as you need to get back on track. This book is also meant to be used as a refresher course, if you need it.

Life Is Not a Dress Rehearsal

While our risk reduction never goes to zero, I truly believe that each of us has the power within to dramatically reduce our personal chances of getting a number of diseases such as type 2 diabetes, heart attack, stroke, various cancers, Alzheimer's, osteo-arthritis, and osteoporosis. Additionally, I know only too well that there are other prevalent diseases, such as rheumatoid arthritis, multiple sclerosis, Parkinson's, and many types of cancer, that do not have preventive solutions at this time. However, in my experience, patients with these diseases often seem to do better if they are at a healthy weight, are physically active, and exercise.

There are no guarantees in life, but you can make a big difference in your health by maintaining a healthy weight, being physically active every day, and exercising (mainly cardio along with some resistance and strength training) consistently three or four times per week. The cost to all of us, and to society in general, of all the lifestyle-induced chronic diseases that we are witnessing world-wide is not sustainable.

Because the Health First program has worked for so many of my patients, I know that it can work for you, too. I wish you every success and look forward to you joining the ranks by becoming a health ambassador through participation in this program.

Afterword

My Life Is Transformed

One patient most kindly took the trouble to write her story for this book. I hope you find it as inspiring as I found it moving.

Being 100 pounds overweight affected every aspect of my life. I tended to sit on the sidelines and watch life go by, rather than participate fully. All physical movement – walking, climbing stairs, bending over, stepping into or out of the bathtub – was difficult and often uncomfortable. I had a constant negative track running in my head, pointing out my faults. Feelings of embarrassment and even humiliation regarding my size were common.

Since I lost those 100 pounds, my health has improved dramatically. My "numbers" (blood pressure, cholesterol, even bone density) are good. My risk of developing certain diseases/conditions has been greatly reduced.

I'm more physically fit. I walk on the treadmill for between thirty-five and fifty minutes (two to three miles) almost daily. This alone has helped me to lead a more active lifestyle. I take a yoga class, which I really enjoy. I'm totally amazed at what my body is able to do in this class. My balance has improved. I can climb stairs easily, no longer having to haul myself up using the handrail. I experience less joint pain. I can reach all my body parts!

My husband and I now enjoy traveling. We actively seek out walking tours in the European cities we visit, and, when arriving in smaller towns, we park the car and set out to explore on foot. I can walk down the aisle of the airplane without squeezing through. I fit in the airplane seat and the seat belt fits with inches to spare.

I can buy clothes in "normal" stores in the petite section – a far cry from the plus-size stores. I drive a Smart car. I'm not sure I would have fit, 100 pounds ago. Also, I would have felt rather silly in such a small car.

I eat out in restaurants comfortably. I fit in the booths (didn't before – had to request a table with chairs). I order what I please (mostly healthy), not fearing what others are thinking.

I have a more positive attitude toward myself and life in general. I'm much more even-tempered. I realize now how angry I was. I experience greater mental clarity. No more "food fog."

I'm more confident. Others do not look at me because of my "fatness." The constant self-deprecating negative track is gone.

My husband and I put a hot tub in our backyard. This means a bathing suit. I do it! (A girlfriend and I went to Greece two years ago. We were celebrating our forty-seven years of friendship, her retirement, my weight loss, and our turning sixty. She asked me if I was taking a bathing suit. I replied that I was. I had sat on the sidelines most of my life and I wasn't going to do that anymore!)

My relationship with my husband has changed. He, too, followed Dr. Hirsch's program, and lost over 80 pounds. I'm not sure how exactly to express the change, but we are much closer. Perhaps it was working so hard together to develop a healthier lifestyle. We appreciate each other more.

I'm very careful with the food I choose and cook. We eat very little prepared food or red meat (huge change). I cook most of our meals from scratch, making all soups, breads, and even yogurt.

I look better – maybe more wrinkled, but better. I feel terrific, energetic, healthy, fit.

I have tried other diets, and I was fine for a time. But the weight was all regained, along with quite a few extra pounds.

With Dr. Hirsch's program, I consistently lost weight – on average 2 pounds a week. I did not have a week when I did not lose something. That kept me motivated to keep going. Of course, I had the huge advantage of seeing Dr. Hirsch face to face every week. His positive support and encouragement kept me going.

For me, the hardest part of the program was getting into an exercise routine. I had led a very sedentary life, so getting up and moving was quite a challenge. I started by walking around the block (well, only a few houses from home at first). As the weather got colder, I walked in the local mall, then on a "manual" treadmill, and now I walk on a programmable electric treadmill.

My lowest point was when my father passed away. I was just a few months into the program. It was somewhat hard to stay focused during that time. Probably the most frustrating time was when I approached the 100-pound point and started losing more slowly.

Most of the people around me, both family and friends, were supportive. My husband was extremely supportive.

Dr. Hirsch's guidelines for healthy eating (food choices, portion control) are clear and uncomplicated. Once you get in the groove of exercising, you'll feel so terrific and have so much energy you'll wonder why it took so long to get moving.

Words cannot express the gratitude both my husband and I feel for Dr. Hirsch and his wonderful, lifesaving program. He patiently coached us, prodded us, and helped us to transform our lives from unhealthy and sedentary to active, healthy, and fully alive. Thank you, thank you, thank you, thank you, Dr. Hirsch!

–KATHY STEWART, a sixty-two-year-old
retired elementary school teacher

Appendix

Health First Food Budget and Snack Times: A Quick Reference

The Table of Threes and Fours				
3 portions per week	**4 portions per week**	**3 portions per day**	**4 portions per day**	**Unlimited servings**
Meat	Eggs	Milk, yogurt, milk alternatives*	Fruit	Vegetables
Fish		Starch (females)	Starch (males)	Poultry**
Cheese*				
*On days you have cheese, you're permitted just 2 portions of milk, yogurt, or milk alternatives.				
**For those without kidney disease.				
Note re: Alcohol				
Females: up to 4 drinks per week				
Males: up to 7 drinks per week				

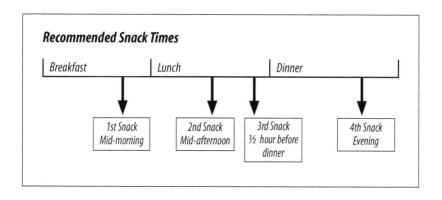

Recommended Snack Times

Breakfast — Lunch — Dinner

- 1st Snack Mid-morning
- 2nd Snack Mid-afternoon
- 3rd Snack ½ hour before dinner
- 4th Snack Evening

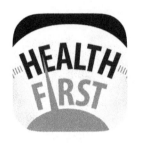

The free HEALTH FIRST App is an amazing coach, enabling you to put into practice everything you've learned in this book. This simple, practical, and powerful App will help you:

- **Keep track of your daily and weekly food budget**

- **And stay mindful of:**
  - your food portions
  - your daily physical activity (steps per day)
  - your exercise for the week

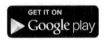

About the Author

Steve Hirsch, MD CCFP FCFP, is passionate about leading a healthy life, which for him includes exercise, proper diet, and daily mindfulness meditation. He has run twenty-four marathons, including five Boston Marathons, and is also an avid cyclist. His other interests include theater, music, and fine dining.

For the last thirty years, Dr. Hirsch has enjoyed a broad-based, comprehensive family medicine practice in the Mississauga/ Oakville area of Ontario, Canada. He is on staff in the Department of Primary Care at Trillium Health Partners, a large community hospital in Mississauga. He is also a lecturer in the Department of Family and Community Medicine at the University of Toronto.

Dr. Hirsch was chief of the Department of Family Medicine at the Credit Valley Hospital for six years, as well as a part-time emergency physician from 1983 to 2006. A graduate of Dalhousie University's Faculty of Medicine and the University of Toronto's Family Medicine Residency program, Dr. Hirsch holds certification and a fellowship with the College of Family Physicians of Canada.

Since 1997, Dr. Hirsch has also been a senior medical consultant with the Medcan Clinic, an executive health-care clinic in Toronto. An accomplished seminar leader, he has conducted seminars for over a decade on health issues in retirement for Retirement Planning Institute, a company based in Ottawa, Ontario.

A long-time resident of Thornhill, Ontario, Dr. Hirsch lives with his wife, Paula, and has two grown sons, Jason and Neil.

CPSIA information can be obtained
at www.ICGtesting.com
Printed in the USA
LVHW051553310719
626020LV00016B/934

plum
PLUS

INTRODUCING THE NEW PLUM PLUS PROGRAM
Join today!

FOR $39 A YEAR, YOU'LL ENJOY THESE MEMBER BENEFITS AND MORE IN-STORE AND ONLINE

Save an extra 10% on almost everything[1]

Earn 5 plum points on almost every dollar spent[2]

Enjoy free shipping everyday[3]

LEARN MORE AT INDIGO.CA/PLUM
IREWARDS MEMBERS CAN CONVERT FOR FREE[4]!

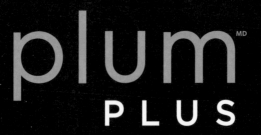

plum^{MD} PLUS

VOICI LE TOUT NOUVEAU PROGRAMME DE RÉCOMPENSES PLUM PLUS

Inscrivez-vous dès aujourd'hui!

POUR SEULEMENT 39 $ PAR ANNÉE, PROFITEZ D'AVANTAGES EXCLUSIFS RÉSERVÉS AUX MEMBRES, EN MAGASIN ET EN LIGNE

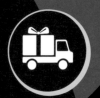

Obtenez un rabais additionnel de 10 % sur la plupart des articles[1]

Recevez 5 points plum pour presque chaque dollar dépensé[2]

Profitez de l'expédition gratuite en tout temps[3]

POUR EN SAVOIR PLUS, VISITEZ INDIGO.CA/PLUM

LES MEMBRES IREWARDS PEUVENT TRANSFÉRER LEUR COMPTE SANS FRAIS ADDITIONNELS[4]!

[1]En vigueur dans les magasins au Canada et à indigo.ca, à l'achat d'articles admissibles, avant les taxes, mais après les rabais applicables et l'échange de points, pour les détenteurs d'un abonnement plum PLUS valide. Les livres numériques, les appareils électroniques et accessoires connexes, les articles de marque American Girl^{MD} (autres que les Wellie Wishers^{MC}), LEGO^{MD}, Shinola et Casper, les Expériences Indigo, les cartes-cadeaux, les abonnements plum PLUS, les frais d'expédition, les produits de la Fondation Indigo pour l'amour de la lecture et les dons faits à celle-ci ne sont pas des articles admissibles. Pour en savoir plus sur le programme, consultez la page indigo.ca/recompenses. [2]Aucun point ne sera attribué pour : les livres numériques, les appareils électroniques, les accessoires connexes, les services American Girl^{MD}, les articles LEGO^{MD} Mindstorms, les abonnements plum PLUS, les cartes-cadeaux, les produits de la Fondation Indigo pour l'amour de la lecture ou les dons faits à celle-ci, les frais d'expédition, l'échange de points lors d'une transaction, les taxes, et toute autre exclusion qui pourrait s'appliquer. Pour en savoir plus sur le programme, consultez la page indigo.ca/recompenses. [3]En vigueur à indigo.ca à l'achat d'articles admissibles, pour les détenteurs d'un abonnement plum PLUS valide. Ne s'applique pas aux articles lourds ou surdimensionnés ni aux expéditions à des endroits éloignés, comme indiqué à indigo.ca/expedition-gratuite. [4]Les membres iRewards peuvent fermer leur compte actuel et transférer leur solde de points lorsqu'ils passent au programme plum PLUS, et ce, sans frais additionnels, pour une période de 12 mois.